AROMATHERAPY
Therapy
BASICS

AROMATHERAPY
Therapy
BASICS

Helen McGuinness

Hodder & Stoughton
A MEMBER OF THE HODDER HEADLINE GROUP

ISBN 0 340 67993X

First published 1997
Impression number   10 9 8 7 6 5 4 3 2 1
Year   2001 2000 1999 1998 1997

The Author and Publisher cannot be held responsible for any misadventure resulting from the misuse of essential oils, or any other therapeutic method mentioned in this book.

Typeset by Wearset, Boldon, Tyne and Wear.
Printed in Great Britain for Hodder & Stoughton Educational, a division of Hodder Headline Plc, 338 Euston Road, London NW1 3BH by the Bath Press, Bath

CONTENTS

ACKNOWLEDGEMENTS

I would like to extend my thanks to my father, Roy for his great skill in producing the illustrations for this book, and to my mother, Valerie for her patience in checking the text for grammar, and especially for her encouragement. My thanks also goes to my husband Mark who has provided considerable help, love and support throughout the development of this book.

My grateful thanks also extends to the following people:

Deirdre Moynihan and Stephanie Mealey of AVCS for their technical help in checking the accuracy of the text and for their valued contributions; John Marks for his technical help with the aroma chemistry chapter; Chris Ockendon of New Horizon Aromatics for his valued contributions to the text; Berni Hephrun of Butterbur and Sage for supplying information regarding the quality of essential oils; Alan Harris, the secretary of the ATC for providing me with valuable information. Finally, thanks are due to all my students at the Holistic Training Centre, Southampton, for their support and encouragement in the development of the book and for their valued contributions.

INTRODUCTION

Aromatherapy has grown in popularity over the past ten years to become recognised as a complementary therapy, and for those interested in holistic health care, it offers a very rewarding career.

This workbook is intended for those undertaking a professional course of training in aromatherapy or for qualified aromatherapists who want to update and extend their knowledge of the subject. It meets the underpinning knowledge requirements of the NVQ Level III in Aromatherapy Massage, but also covers the knowledge requirements of more traditional diploma courses.

The material contained within the book has been designed to be interactive. Each chapter has tasks and self-assessment questions to complete, in order to assess overall understanding of the individual subject areas.

As well as providing a comprehensive knowledge of aromatherapy, the aim of the workbook is to help candidates to generate portfolio evidence of underpinning knowledge for their NVQ qualification.

Chapter 1

INTRODUCTION TO AROMATHERAPY

Aromatherapy is the art of using essential oils to help restore balance in the body, and is a form of natural healing which is more than 8,000 years old. Today it represents one of the fastest growing complementary therapies in the UK.

- A competent aromatherapist needs to be able to understand aromatherapy as a holistic therapy, in order to apply suitable treatments, and give accurate advice and guidance to clients.

By the end of this chapter you will be able to relate the following knowledge to your practical work carried out as an aromatherapist:

- how aromatherapy has developed
- uses of aromatherapy.

Aromatherapy is a truly holistic therapy, as it aims to treat the whole person by taking account not only of their physical state but also their emotions, which can have a profound effect on general well-being. It works on the principle that the most effective way to promote health and prevent illness is to strengthen the body's immune system; in so doing, it helps to restore the harmony between mind and body.

The primary form of aromatherapy applications involves using essential oils in the following ways:

- topically to the skin via massage, diluted in a carrier oil
- inhalations
- compresses
- aromatic baths.

An essential oil is the highly concentrated volatile substance obtained from various parts of the aromatic plant.

Disillusionment with orthodox medicine has caused many people to turn to the natural remedies that have been part of our folklore for many thousands of years.

THE HISTORY OF AROMATHERAPY

The history of the application of essential oils to the human body goes back to at least 2,000 BC. Records in the Bible show the use of plants and their aromatic oils both for the treatment of illness and for religious purposes.

The first evidence of the wide-ranging use of aromatic oils comes from Ancient Egypt – Egyptians extracted oils by a method of infusion, and used them as cosmetics. One of the most famous Egyptian aromatic formulas was a mixture of 16 aromatic substances called 'kyphi' which was later used as a perfume by the Greeks and Romans. One of the earliest uses of aromatic oils by the Egyptians was incense for religious purposes and for embalming the dead to delay decomposition of bodies.

The ancient Greeks and Romans acquired much of their knowledge regarding the use of aromatics oils from the Egyptians. The Greek, Herodotus, was the first person to record the method of distillation of turpentine, around 425 BC.

The Greeks and Romans used aromatic oils for aromatic massages and in daily baths. They discovered that the odour of certain plants and flowers was stimulating and invigorating, while others were sedative and relaxing. The Greek soldiers also carried essential oil such as myrrh into battle with them for the treatment of wounds. Hippocrates, a Greek physician, wrote about a vast range of medicinal plants, and claimed that the best way to achieve good health was to have an aromatic bath and scented massage every day!

The writings of Hippocrates and others were translated into Arabic languages; after the fall of Rome and the advent of Christianity, surviving Roman physicians fled to Constantinople, taking their books and knowledge with them.

The most famous Arab physician was Avicenna, who reputedly wrote over 100 books describing over 800 plants and their effects on the body. However, his most important act in terms of aromatherapy is being credited with inventing the refrigerated coil, a development of the more primitive form of distillation, which he used to produce pure oils and aromatic waters.

The earliest written record of the use of aromatic oils in England was in the 13th century. From 1470–1670, the invention and development of printing across Europe resulted in the publication of many herbals or books which included recipes for making essential oils. It is a known fact that people who used aromatic oils were the only ones to survive the Plague which struck Europe during these centuries, due to the fact that the vast majority of essential oils have antiseptic properties.

The knowledge of the *medicinal* properties of plants was later reinforced by Nicholas Culpeper, a celebrated herbalist who wrote a book of herbs in 1652 which contained the medicinal properties of hundreds of plants.

MODERN DEVELOPMENTS

The *scientific* study of the therapeutic properties of essential oils was commenced by the French cosmetic chemist, Renee Gattefosse, in the 1920s. He discovered through burning his arm while making fragrances in his laboratory, that the essential oil of lavender was exceptionally healing to the skin, and left no scarring. This discovery led him to undertake a great deal of research into the medicinal uses of essential oils, and his work revealed that it is possible for essential oils to penetrate the skin and be carried in the blood and lymphatic system to the organs.

Other French doctors and scientists continued his work and helped to validate the status of essential oils as scientific substances. Most notably, Dr Jean Valnet used essential oils to treat severe burns and battle injuries, in the absence of medical supplies. His book *Aromatherapie* (translated as *The Practice of Aromatherapy*) confirms the findings of Gattefosse, and has become an established textbook among serious aromatherapy practitioners.

Despite this however, herbal medicine and aromatic remedies lost credibility with the growth of modern synthetic drug industry. By the middle of the 20th century, the role of essential oils was reduced to being employed in the perfumes, cosmetic and food industry.

AROMATHERAPY IN BRITAIN

The term 'aromatherapy' was coined by Gattefosse, and was introduced to Britain in the late 1950s by Marguerite Maury, who was a student of Gattefosse. She developed Gattefosse's work to a more practical conclusion, by combining the use of essential oils with massage. She developed specialised massage techniques and the 'individual prescription', a more holistic approach in which essences are chosen according to the physical and emotional needs of the client. Marguerite Maury devoted the rest of her working life to teaching and training therapists in the special techniques she had developed. Her first lectures in Britain were to beauty therapists, who began to introduce essential oils with massage to help relieve stress and skin conditions.

Today, thanks to Marguerite Maury, aromatherapy has developed from being used mainly in perfumes and cosmetics, to a more holistic treatment – true aromatherapy lies in selecting and blending oils individually for each client. But, despite its ancient origins, aromatherapy is still in its infancy in this country. Research into this fascinating therapy is still taking place, as it becomes recognised as a complementary therapy, and is used in many hospitals and clinics across the country.

Aromatherapy today represents a de-stressing programme for the whole person and its extensive uses may complement orthodox treatments to help restore the body's balance. May this wonderful therapy continue to soothe our stressed lives and progress well into the 21st century.

☞ TASK

Research an aspect of aromatherapy that interests you and report your findings. You may wish to consider the following:

- Is aromatherapy being used locally in your chosen aspect of research? If so, where and how?
- How long has aromatherapy been used in this area?
- How effective has aromatherapy been in this area?
- Have any particular essential oils been found to be most effective?
- If aromatherapy is not being used in your area of interest, is there a possible business opportunity?

❓ SELF-ASSESSMENT QUESTIONS

1. Define the term 'aromatherapy'.

....

....

....

....

2. Why is aromatherapy often referred to as a 'holistic therapy'?

....

....

....

3. Give a brief outline of how aromatherapy developed from its more primitive use in Egyptian times to become a complementary therapy today.

....

....

....

....

....

....

....

....

....

....

....

....

....

....

....

....

....

....

....

Chapter 2

SAFETY IN AROMATHERAPY

Essential oils have been used in the form of the whole plant for thousands of years for medicinal and cosmetic purposes, but when distilled from the plant they become a hundred times more concentrated. Their physical, physiological and pharmacological effects on the body are therefore increased, and knowledge of safe levels of usage are of paramount important to a practising aromatherapist. *Proportion* is the key to a safe aromatherapy practice.

- A competent aromatherapist needs to understand and apply all safety precautions to the use of essential oils, to ensure a safe and effective treatment.

By the end of this chapter you will be able to relate the following knowledge to your work as an aromatherapist:

- contra-indications to aromatherapy ✓
- hazards associated with essential oils
- safety precautions and guidelines when practising aromatherapy
- storage and safe handling of essential oils.

As the benefits of aromatherapy are generally so far reaching, it is tempting to assume that it will be effective for everyone. However, there are certain medical conditions which may contra-indicate treatment or cases that may require special care and handling.

Contra-indications may be classified in the following way:

- general contra-indications which affect all treatments
- those that are localised and which affect specific areas
- those which require special care.

> ## KEY NOTE
>
> For insurance purposes and in order to work within strict ethical guidelines, an aromatherapist must ensure that if a client is currently undergoing medical treatment or is under hospital care, then approval is sought from the client's GP before any form of treatment is undertaken.
>
> If you are in any doubt about the suitability of your client for aromatherapy treatments, always seek approval from the client's GP before commencing treatment.

CONTRA-INDICATIONS TO AROMATHERAPY TREATMENTS

- *Severe circulatory disorders and heart conditions*   general contra-indication: GP referral
- *History of thrombosis or embolism*   general contra-indication: GP referral
- *High or low blood pressure*   general contra-indication: GP referral
- *Epilepsy*   general contra-indication: GP referral
- *Diabetes*   general contra-indication: GP referral
- *Dysfunction of the nervous system*   general contra-indication: GP referral
- *Any potentially fatal condition (ie cancer)*   general contra-indication: GP/hospital referral
- *Fever*   general contra-indication
- *Migraine*   some strong odours may exacerbate an attack: special care required
- *Recent operations, fractures and sprains*   localised contra-indication
- *Severe bruising in the treatment area*   localised contra-indication
- *Recent haemorrhaging or swelling*   localised contra-indication: may require GP referral, depending on severity of haemorrhage
- *Over varicose veins*   localised contra-indication
- *Skin disorders*   localised contra-indication (general contra-indication if infected or infectious)
- *Open cuts, abrasions and scar tissue*   localised contra-indication (general contra-indication if infected)
- *Allergies and skin intolerances*   requires special care and handling: carry out skin test and avoid all essential oils known to be skin irritants or sensitisers
- *Pregnancy*   requires special care and handling: use lower dilution of oils

and avoid all toxic oils. May require GP referral if there are any
complications with the pregnancy
- *Medication*   GP referral
- *Children and babies*   require special care and handling: use lower dilution
  of oils and avoid all toxic oils
- *Homeopathic preparations*   requires special care and handling: refer to
  Homeopath as some strong odours may antidote homeopathic
  preparations

KEY NOTE

Essential oils which are considered to be safe to use during pregnancy in
a lower dilution (ie 1%) include:

Bergamot, Chamomile (Roman and German)*, Cypress,
Frankincense*, Geranium, Grapefruit, Lavender*, Lemon, Mandarin,
Neroli, Orange, Patchouli, Petitgrain, Rose otto*, Sandalwood and
Ylang Ylang.

*   Avoid during first few months of pregnancy

The majority of essential oils when used correctly in aromatherapy treatments
represent a negligible risk. However it should be remembered that essential
oils are very powerful and concentrated substances, and should therefore be
employed with a great deal of care as inappropriate use may cause undesired
effects.

There are three main types of hazards associated with essential oils:

- toxicity
- irritation
- sensitisation.

TOXICITY

Toxicity is a broad term which is used in aromatherapy to describe the
hazardous effects associated with the misuse of essential oils.

There are two main categories of toxicity:

- acute
- chronic.

ACUTE TOXICITY

This refers to the result of a short-term administration of a substance, and usually involves a single high lethal dose. Acute toxicity may be sub-categorised into the following classifications:

- *Acute oral toxicity* – this literally means 'poisoning' when an essential oil is taken orally in a high lethal dose; this may result in death.
- *Acute dermal toxicity* – high levels of essential oils are applied and readily absorbed through the skin to cause systemic toxicity, which could cause damage to the liver and kidneys (these are the two major organs of the body to filter out unwanted toxic substances from the bloodstream).

CHRONIC TOXICITY

This is the repeated use of a substance over a period of weeks, months or years, and is used to describe the adverse effects produced in the skin or elsewhere in the body, either by external or internal use.

Adverse effects of chronic toxicity may include headaches, nausea, minor skin eruptions, and lethargy.

━━━━ KEY NOTE ━━━━

The degree of toxicity in aromatherapy depends not only on the amount of essential oils used but also on its route of administration. Oral administration represents by far the highest risk of toxicity and therefore should NOT be used in aromatherapy unless under the direction of a qualified Medical Practitioner.

It should be noted that external use of essential oils is the only established form of treatment in the UK at this present time.

As toxicity is dose-dependent, the only risk of toxicity with essential oils is concerned with overuse and overdose.

Dose-dependency also refers to the size of the individual being treated: special care is required when treating a baby or young child as they are much more likely to develop toxicity with a much smaller amount of essential oil than an adult.

Common examples of toxic essential oils include:

- Aniseed
- Arnica
- Mugwort

- Pennyroyal
- Sassafras
- Savory
- Thuja
- Wintergreen
- Wormwood.

PHOTOTOXICITY

This term refers to a photochemical reaction which takes place in the skin by the combination of a phototoxic oil and ultra-violet rays. It may result in a mild colour change, to rapid tanning and hyper pigmentation. Depending on the severity of the photochemical reaction, it may cause blistering or deep weeping burns.

The most common phototoxic agents in essential oils are *furocoumarins* (such as bergaptene in bergamot oil) which upon exposure to sunlight (natural or artificial) can cause adverse skin reactions.

Common examples of essential oils which may present a risk of phototoxicity include:

- Bergamot (expressed – a method of production for citrus oils in which oil is expressed from the rind of the fruit)
- Lemon (expressed)
- Bitter Orange (expressed)
- Lime (expressed)
- Grapefruit (expressed)

The risk of phototoxicity can be eliminated or at least reduced to safe levels by adhering to the following safe practice:

- Use furocoumarin free bergamot (FCF) (see Key Note below) or distilled citrus oils which are non-phototoxic.
- Use sunscreen to reduce the potential effect of phototoxicity.
- Ensure that the area treated is covered and is not exposed to strong sunlight (natural or artificial) for at least eight hours following treatment with phototoxic oils.

————— KEY NOTE —————

Bergamot is an example of a fractionated essential oil (ie, one that has part of the chemical composition removed). Research has shown that bergamot containing less than one part per 1,000 of bergaptene (the substance known to cause phototoxicity) is safe to use on the skin. Bergamot FCF indicates that the phototoxic bergaptene has been removed or reduced to a safe level to use on the skin.

IRRITATION

This is the most common type of reaction of the skin to essential oils, and is caused when a substance such as an essential oil reacts with the mast cells of the skin and releases histamine.

The term *irritation* refers to localised inflammation which may affect the skin and mucous membranes, and results in itchiness as well as varying degrees of inflammation.

Irritation is dose-dependent, and so reaction is directly proportional to the amount used in treatment.

—————— K E Y   N O T E ——————

The risk of irritation is most acute when essential oils are used undiluted or are used in high concentration. It is interesting to note that there appears to be a wide tolerance variation between individuals. Reactions are idiosyncratic (they only affect a small majority of people).

As the mucous membranes are thinner and much more fragile than the skin, they are in danger of becoming irritated. Care must be taken with the amount of essential oil used for inhalations (due to the risk of irritating the respiratory tract). Essential oils should never be used via the rectum, vagina or mouth, due to their potential risk of irritation to the mucous membrane of the urino-genital and alimentary tract organs. Essential oils should be kept well away from the eyes.

Common examples of essential oils representing a risk of irritation include:

- Cinnamon Leaf
- Clove Bud
- Clove Stem
- Clove Leaf
- Red Thyme
- Wild Thyme.

Note: Some more common essential oils may occasionally cause irritation if used undiluted on the skin.

SENSITISATION

This is an allergic reaction to an essential oil, and usually takes the form of a rash, similar to the reaction of the skin to urticaria. For sensitisation to occur, the allergen (ie an essential oil) must penetrate the skin and will involve an immune response by the release of histamine. It will cause an inflammatory reaction, brought about by the cells of the immune system (T-lymphocytes) becoming sensitised. Upon first exposure to the substance, the effects on the skin will be slight if at all; but on repeated application of the same substance, the immune system will produce a reaction similar to dermal inflammation and the skin may appear blotchy and irritated.

Sensitisation is not dose-dependent, and so it is not dependent on concentration. Intolerance may build up on repeated contact with a sensitising oil, or after one application.

Common examples of essential oils which may cause sensitisation include:

- Cinnamon (bark, leaf and stem)
- Ginger
- Lemon
- Lemongrass
- Lime
- Melissa
- Bitter Orange
- Peppermint
- Teatree
- Thyme.

——————— KEY NOTE ———————

When dealing with clients with sensitive skin or skin with intolerances, it is wise to perform a patch test for both irritation and sensitisation of a potentially hazardous oil.

In order to test for irritation, apply a couple of drops of the essential oil to the inside of a plaster, place on the inside of the forearm and leave unwashed for 24 hours. Repeat the test a second time if you wish to test for sensitisation.

Prior to working on areas such as the face and neck where cosmetics have been used, it is advisable to ensure that all preparations have been removed before applying essential oils, due to the risk of cross-sensitisation occurring on areas which are building up sensitivity to cosmetics. A positive result (which may indicate irritation) may result in erythema, itching and swelling. For female clients, skin sensitivity generally increases just before a menstrual period and at ovulation, due to hormonal influences at this time.

SAFETY PRECAUTIONS WHEN USING ESSENTIAL OILS

When using essential oils, the following safety precautions should be followed to ensure a safe, effective treatment with no adverse effects to either the client or the therapist:

- Always work in a well ventilated area.
- Keep and dispense essential oils away from the treatment area, preferably in a separate room.
- In between clients, air the treatment room and allow yourself a break of at least five minutes.
- Keep essential oils away from eyes and other sensitive parts of the face.
- Always undertake a detailed consultation to ascertain a client's physical and psychological condition, along with any medication they may be taking.
- If your client presents a medical condition, always refer them to their GP before treating.
- Never take essential oils by mouth, rectum or vagina, unless under medical instructions.
- Never apply undiluted oils to the skin.
- Always use in sensible proportions.
- Avoid prolonged use of the same essential oil.
- If your client suffers with sensitive skin or allergies, it is advisable to carry out a simple skin test before using an essential oil for the first time.
- Always label all blends.
- Always keep a full and accurate record of the essential oils used on a client and their dilution.
- Never use an essential oil with which you are not familiar.

SAFE HANDLING AND STORAGE

Due to the fact that essential oils are concentrated substances and are toxic if misused, great care must be taken when storing and handling them:

- Store in dark glass bottles in normal to cool temperatures (approx. 65° Fahrenheit/18° Centigrade), with lids secured tightly to prevent evaporation.
- Store all essential oils out of the reach of children.
- Keep essential oils away from naked flames, as they are highly flammable.
- Take care when handling essential oil bottles to ensure that your skin does not come into contact with the undiluted oil, and that you avoid transferring it from your hands to more sensitive parts (ie, nose, face and neck).
- Wash hands thoroughly in between clients, to remove as much of the oil as possible.
- Avoid using oils if your skin is cracked and sore.

All essential oils sold for professional and home use should carry safety precautions in their labelling.

An independent body, the Aromatherapy Trade Council (ATC), was formed in 1992 by responsible essential oils suppliers. Its aims are to:

- help raise standards and offer protection to the consumer
- establish guidelines for safety, labelling and packaging of essential oils
- establish standards of quality in essential oils and aromatherapy products
- promote the responsible use of aromatherapy products.

The Code of Practice recommended by the ATC includes the following:

- Integral single drop dispensers are to be incorporated in all bottles of essential oil on sale to the general public.
- The following warnings are to be printed on the label:
  * instructions for use: add up to 5 drops of essential oil to 10 ml of carrier, for instance
  * keep away from children and delicate areas such as the eyes
  * do not apply undiluted to the skin
  * do not take internally
  * the quantity of essential oil in the bottle (5 ml, 10 ml, 12 ml for instance)
  * the company's name and address.

━━━━━━━━━━ **K E Y N O T E** ━━━━━━━━━━

In order to comply with consumer legislation, essential oils suppliers have a duty to carry out responsible marketing.

The Medicines Act 1968 clearly states that no medicinal claims can be made on labels, promotional material or advertisements regarding products that have not been licensed. This means that no aromatherapy product can make remedial claims if it relates to a specific disease or adverse condition.

TASK

Complete the following table to identify the type of hazard associated with essential oils.

TABLE 1: *Hazards associated with essential oils*

Hazard	Description
	Essential oil taken orally in a high lethal dose; can be fatal.
	High levels of essential oils are applied to skin, and cause systemic toxicity; affects liver and kidneys.
	Photochemical reaction which takes place in skin by combination of phototoxic oil and ultra-violet rays.
	Localised inflammation of skin, caused by essential oil reacting with the mast cells of skin releasing histamine. Affects skin and mucous membrane and is dose-dependent.
	Allergic reaction to an essential oil, involves an immune response by releasing histamine and causes the T-lymphocytes to become sensitised. Reaction may be slight on first exposure to allergen but on repeated exposure skin may appear blotchy and irritated. Is not dose-dependent.

SELF-ASSESSMENT QUESTIONS

1. Why is safety an important factor when using essential oils?

   ....

   ....

   ....

2. State ten safety precautions to be taken into account when practising aromatherapy.

....

....

....

....

....

....

....

....

....

....

3. State five conditions which may contra-indicate aromatherapy treatment, stating the action required in each case.

....

....

....

....

....

....

....

....

4. State five safety factors to be taken into account when storing essential oils.

....

....

....

....

....

5. State five essential oils which are unsafe to use in aromatherapy.

....

....

....

....

....

6. List five safety factors which should be on the label of essential oil bottles sold for professional and home use.

....

....

....

....

....

Chapter 3

~

THE EXTRACTION OF AN ESSENTIAL OIL

The most important ingredient in aromatherapy is the essential oil, a highly concentrated volatile substance obtained from various parts of the aromatic plant. Despite being used extensively in the food industry as flavourings and in the cosmetic industry in perfumes, when used in aromatherapy they have the ability to penetrate the skin and be absorbed into the bloodstream. Utmost care must therefore be taken in their application to the body.

- A competent aromatherapist must know the nature and effects of essential oils in order to understand the physical and psychological effects of aromatherapy treatments.

By the end of this chapter you will be able to relate the following knowledge to your work as an aromatherapist:

- the nature and origins of essential oils
- methods of extracting essential oils
- factors to consider when storing essential oils
- common forms of adulteration
- factors to consider when purchasing essential oils
- vocabulary associated with an essential oil.

Essential oils play an important role in the plant, as they are responsible for their fragrance and are the most concentrated part of its vital force or energy. A typical essential oil consists of over 100 organic chemical compounds which influence its aroma, therapeutic effects and in certain cases its potential hazards (such as irritation, sensitisation or toxicity).

Essential oils are present in the plant in special cells, and may be extracted from various parts of the plant matter; for example, the leaves, flowers, fruit, grass, roots, wood, bark, gums and blossom.

Essential oils are usually present in minute quantities in comparison to the mass of the whole plant, and may exist in the plant material in concentrations ranging from 0.01 to 10 per cent.

The nature of essential oils are therefore complex as they exhibit the following various characteristics:

- *Highly concentrated*   when extracted from the raw material, an essential oil can become 100 times more concentrated
- *Highly aromatic*   the individual aroma of the essential oil becomes more defined after being extracted from the plant
- *Highly volatile*   they evaporate quickly on contact with the air
- *Liquid*   most are liquid, although some are solid at room temperature (eg, rose)
- *Mainly colourless or pale yellow*   although some are more obviously coloured (eg, blue chamomile)
- *Insoluble in water*   they will only dissolve in alcohols, fats, oils and waxes.

--- **KEY NOTE** ---

Due to their sensitivity, it is advisable to store essential oils in a cool, dark place away from heat and light to protect against the damaging effects of ultra-violet light.

Storing essential oils in dark green bottles with lids tightly secured, will help prevent oxidation and degradation.

Remember that the more air that is allowed into the essential oil bottle, the more rapidly oxidation will take place.

METHODS OF EXTRACTION

As essential oils are extracts from plant, they are subject to several processes and can vary according to:

- where they are grown
- the climate

- the altitude
- the soil
- the agricultural methods
- the time of harvesting.

It is therefore very important that the starting material used to produce the essential oil represents the natural biochemistry of the plant, in order that an oil with the highest grade of quality may be produced.

Due to their differences in distribution there are several methods of producing essential oils:

- steam distillation
- solvent extraction
- expression
- enfleurage
- super-critical carbon dioxide extraction
- phytonic process.

STEAM DISTILLATION

This is the oldest and most established method of extracting the essential oil from the plant. Plant material such as flowers and leaves need very little preparation prior to being distilled, except that they need to be cut up to allow the cell walls of the plant to rupture and the volatile oil to escape.

- The process involves placing the prepared plant material, such as leaves and flowers, into a large stainless steel container called a *still*.
- Steam is then passed under pressure through the plant material, and the heat causes the globules of essential oil to burst open, and the oil quickly evaporates.
- The steam and the essential oil vapour then passes out from the top of the still and along a glass tube which is water-cooled, in order to condense the water back into a liquid.
- It is then a relatively simple process to separate the essential oil from the water, since the two do not mix. The water distillate left after extraction of the essential oil is a valuable by-product, and is used as a flower water or hydrolat.

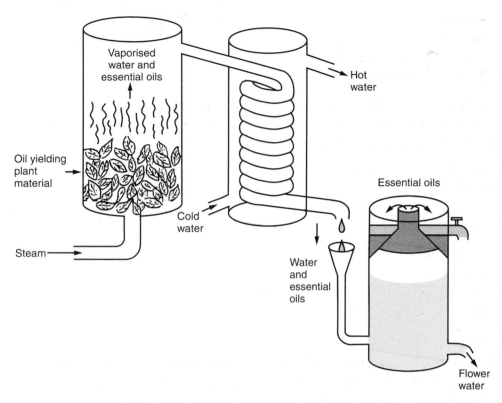

Figure 1
Steam distillation of essential oils

KEY NOTE

During the distillation process, only the very small molecules can evaporate, and it is *these* tiny molecules that constitute the essential oil.

The heat and water used in the distillation process are potentially harmful to the fragile chemical constituents of the essential oil, and can alter the quality of the original plant material. Using low pressure steam and heat, pure water and fresh materials during the distillation process can therefore ensure the production of the best quality and 'environmentally friendly' essential oil.

SOLVENT EXTRACTION

This process involves placing the plant material in a vessel and covering it with a volatile solvent such as petroleum ether, benzene or hexane, which is used to extract the odoriferous part of the material.

- The mixture is slowly heated and the solution is filtered off, resulting in a dark coloured paste called a *concrete* (this is a combination of wax and essential oil or a resinous substance containing resin).
- The concrete then undergoes a second process, when it is agitated with alcohol and chilled in order to recover most of the aromatic liquid and remove the plant waxes.
- The alcohol is then evaporated leaving a high quality flower oil or absolute.

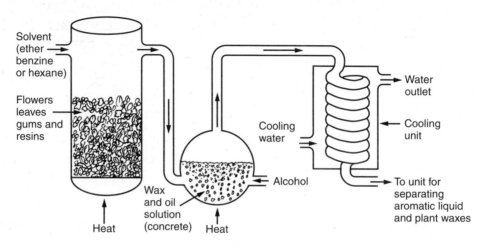

Figure 2
Solvent extraction

KEY NOTE

Solvent extraction is used extensively in the perfumery industry and produces some of the finest flower fragrances. There is an element of controversy regarding the suitability of the use of absolutes in aromatherapy, as they contain solvent residues which may cause adverse skin reactions.

EXPRESSION

This process is used solely for the citrus family and therefore may be used for what may more accurately be called *essences*.

- The oil from the citrus fruit lies in little sacs under the surface of the rind and simply needs to be pressed out.
- The process of expression used to be carried out by hand, where the rind

was literally squeezed by hand until the oil glands in the rind burst. This was then collected in a sponge and squeezed into a container once the sponge was saturated.

- Expression is now carried out by machinery in a process known as *scarification*, and is usually produced in a factory which produces fruit juice in order to maximise the profit from the whole fruit.

KEY NOTE

As no heat is used in the process of expression, the aroma and the delicate chemical structure of the essence extracted is almost identical to that contained within the rind of the fruit.

ENFLEURAGE

This is the traditional method used to extract the finest quality essences from delicate flowers such as rose and jasmine which continue to generate oil after harvesting. It is a very long labour-intensive process, and hence is virtually obsolete now.

- The process involves using wooden glass rectangular frames and spreading a thin layer of purified fat onto the glass.
- Freshly picked petals are then sprinkled over the fat and the glass sheet frames are stacked in tiers. The essence from the flower is then absorbed into the fat.
- The faded petals are removed after 24 hours, after which fresh petals are laid over the fat.
- The process is repeated until the fat is saturated with enough essence from the flower – at this stage it is known as a *pommade*.
- The pommade is then diluted in alcohol to obtain the extracts, and the alcohol evaporates, leaving only the oil. The remaining fat is used commercially to make soap.

Less than 10% of essential oils are produced by this method and enfleurage has been largely replaced by solvent extraction.

SUPER-CRITICAL CARBON DIOXIDE EXTRACTION

This is a relatively new method of extracting essential oils and uses compressed carbon dioxide at very high pressure to extract the essential oil from the plant material.

The essential oils produced by this method are reputed to be of exceptional quality and to be more like the essential oil from the plant in terms of their quality and stability. The disadvantage with using this method is that the equipment used is not only massive, but also extremely expensive to use.

THE PHYTONIC PROCESS

This is a newly developed method of extracting essential oils from the plant, which uses environmentally friendly solvents which have the ability to capture the aromatic oils of the plants at or below room temperature. This ensures that the highly fragile and heat sensitive constituents of the essential oil are neither lost nor altered due to their extraction process. The oils produced by this method are known as 'phytol' oils.

ADULTERATION OF ESSENTIAL OILS

Unfortunately, due to the widespread popularity of essential oils, there is an increased practice of adulteration. Adulterations may take one of several forms:

- A very small quantity of the essential oils may be diluted in a spirit base and therefore is 'let down'.
- A quantity of the main chemical constituent may be added to the essential oils to 'stretch' it; for example, linalool is commonly added to clary sage, lavender, neroli and rosewood.
- Synthetic aromatic substances may be added, resulting in a fabricated oil.
- An essential oil from a cheaper plant may be added, for example, lemon to bergamot or citronella to melissa.
- Some of the chemical constituents may be removed; these oils are known as *fractionated* oils. For example, a main chemical constituent of essential oils such as terpenes can be removed, which is useful for the perfume industry.

KEY NOTE

Essential oils have a highly complex chemistry which makes it impossible to reproduce them synthetically. Synthetic substances or reconstructed oils are in general very successful for perfumery and may also have specific uses in flavourings and pharmaceuticals, but in aromatherapy, essential oils are designed for vibrational healing and therefore it cannot be stressed highly enough that only the *purest* oils in their natural state will give the desired therapeutic effects. Remember that the greater the interference with the chemical constituents of the essential oil, the fewer therapeutic effects it will have. Adulterated oils can have undesired effects such as causing skin irritation and sensitisation.

FACTORS TO CONSIDER WHEN PURCHASING ESSENTIAL OILS

It is imperative to buy essential oils from a reputable supplier. Factors to consider when making your choice include:

Quality

The plant itself, its harvest method, the type of soil used and the country of origin will all play a part in the final determination of quality. If you are in doubt about the quality of an oil, it is advisable to ask suppliers for information concerning the origins of the oil and methods used to test for purity.

KEY NOTE

A supplier or importer of essential oils may use a method of testing for purity called Gas Liquid Chromatography, which is an accurate method of determining an oil's composition, and will reflect the chemical profile of the essential oil. It is often referred to as 'chemical fingerprinting' and is carried out on behalf of some essential oil companies in laboratories by specialist chemists.

Gas Liquid Chromatography will also highlight any undesirable substances such as trace contaminants in the plant such as biocides, herbicides or pesticides which have been used in its production.

Each essential oil tested is given a certification of conformity and a batch number to confirm its purity, if it meets the stringent laboratory tests.

Purity

A pure essential oil can be defined as one which has been produced from a botanical source and has not been modified in any way that alters its unique qualities.

KEY NOTE

Reputable professional suppliers will take steps to ensure that the essential oils they produce are grown by organic means (ie, without the use of chemical fertilisers and poisonous sprays). Organic producers meeting the required standards of production are awarded certificates by the Soil Association in Britain.

Price

In general, the price of an essential oil reflects the yield of oil in the plant along with its production costs. Rose petals produce very little oil, which makes the essential oil fairly expensive, whereas eucalyptus gives a high yield and is relatively cheap. Price is not, however, an indication of purity or quality.

Odour

This will be dependent on the origin of the oil, its method of production and other factors concerning the oil such as storage, transport method, temperature, purity, age, quality and degree of nasal perception.

Best before date

This is important as essential oils are affected by age, light, heat and oxidation. It is useful to know either the production date or its expiry date, to assess its life expectancy to an aromatherapist.

KEY NOTE

As most essential oils are affected by age, it is recommended that they are used within two years of first opening to avoid degradation. Citrus oils have a relatively short life and under good storage conditions will remain unchanged for up to a year.

Despite this, some essential oils such as patchouli actually improve with age, and can remain unchanged for many years.

It is also worth considering that once produced, essential oils have a rather convoluted journey before reaching you, therefore a best before date is very useful in practice.

Origin

The part of the plant used and the country of production may reflect differences in essential oils such as composition, quality or price. Good suppliers' price lists will indicate the part or parts of the plant used to produce the oil along with its country of origin. Remember that the origin of the plant determines its character and chemical composition.

Botanical name of plant

As there are many species or variations of plants, which all exhibit different characteristics, it is important to know the botanical or Latin names of the plant to ensure their authenticity and original character and composition.

Safety

Choose essential oils bottles with child resistant closures.

— K E Y N O T E —

The best advice is to purchase your essential oils from a reputable professional supplier who is prepared to give you as much information as possible regarding the nature of the oils and their origins.

Most professional suppliers list a batch number on the essential oil bottle which is useful to note when you want a repeat order of the same oil.

Although purity is high on the list of priorities when purchasing essential oils, it should be noted that there are no tests, including Gas Liquid Chromatography, which guarantee purity. Whilst Gas Chromatography will highlight any chemical imbalances in the oil which could not be possible in the natural essential oil, it cannot assess its exact chemistry as the precise chemical constituents of essential oils are still largely unknown.

Current EC Regulations are moving towards greater definition and more detailed information regarding the nature of essential oils in order that the consumer may expect to get:

- an essential oil or aromatic from a named botanical source and from a given origin
- an oil which has been tested and analysed by experts who can determine its quality.

TASK

Complete the following table to identify the following terms used in connection with essential oils.

TABLE 2: *Terms used to describe essential oils*

Term	Description
	Aromatic material (viscous or semi-solid perfume material) extracted from plants using solvent extraction.
	Solid or semi-solid dark coloured paste; a combination of wax and essential oil.
	Volatile and aromatic liquid obtained by distillation or expression.
	A by-product of steam distillation.
	Solid or semi-solid natural product, may be prepared or natural (ie exudations from trees).

SELF-ASSESSMENT QUESTIONS

1. Define an essential oil.

   ....

   ....

   ....

2. State five characteristics of an essential oil.

   ....

   ....

   ....

   ....

   ....

3. Why should essential oils never be used in their undiluted form?

....

....

....

4. Give a brief outline of the following methods of extracting essential oils:
   i) steam distillation

....

....

....

....

....

....

....

ii) solvent extraction

....

....

....

....

....

....

....

5. State five important factors to consider when purchasing essential oils.

....

....

....

....

....

6. State three common forms of adulteration of essential oils.

....

....

....

....

....

....

Chapter 4

THE ESSENTIAL OILS

Essential oils have many chemical components which reflect the life force of the plant, and they possess a variety of functions in the plant from which they are derived. These varied functions found within the oil are elements which in the plant form help to fight disease, stimulate growth and reproduction. It is not therefore unreasonable or illogical to expect those same elements to have a variety of functions on the human body.

Orthodox drugs are often very specific and have a single active principle, which is either isolated from the plant or synthetically constructed in a laboratory. Essential oils, however, are more holistic, as they work on several levels.

* A competent aromatherapist needs to know the therapeutic effect attributed to essential oils, to understand their effects on the body.

By the end of this chapter you will be able to relate the following knowledge to your work as an aromatherapist:

* the origin, method of production and therapeutic properties of 30 common essential oils
* vocabulary used to describe the therapeutic properties of essential oils.

As you begin to study the many therapeutic effects of essential oils, you will begin to realise that each oil may be used to treat a variety of conditions, and that most conditions will respond positively to a number of oils.

Essential oils are diverse – there is a large spread of actions with many oils and a degree of overlap in the choice of oil for a particular condition. This is because of the complex chemistry of an essential oil. The chemical constituents of an essential oil are often closely related in their molecular structure to those of human cells and tissues and hormones: therefore, as well as having a direct action upon specific bacteria and viruses, the oils also act by stimulating and reinforcing the body's own defence mechanism.

DIFFERENT TYPES OF ESSENTIAL OIL
BASIL (SWEET)

SUMMARY

A very effective oil, well known for its cephalic property and its effects on digestive and respiratory problems.

Botanical name: *Ocimum Basilicum*
Plant family: Labiatae family
Aroma: very light, clear and sweet but slightly spicy
Colour: colourless or pale yellow
Method of production: steam distillation from the leaves and flowering tops of the plant
Main countries of production: France, Italy, Egypt, Bulgaria, Hungary and the USA

Therapeutic properties:

- analgesic
- antiseptic
- antispasmodic
- carminative
- cephalic
- stomachic
- expectorant
- febrifuge
- nervine
- tonic
- stimulates the adrenal cortex
- antidepressant
- emmenagogue.

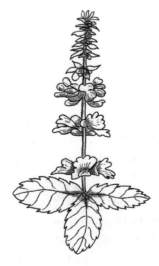

Figure 3
Basil (sweet)

Therapeutic uses:

- muscular aches and pains
- respiratory problems (bronchitis, coughs, colds, asthma and flu)
- digestive problems (gastric spasms, nausea, vomiting, dyspepsia, hiccups)
- nervous tension
- anxiety
- depression
- fatigue (mental and physical)
- headaches
- migraine
- irregular periods
- menstrual pain
- skin care – congested skins and acne
- poor circulation.

Precautions:

- May cause sensitisation and irritation
- Avoid during pregnancy
- There has been recent concern over the carcinogenic effects of methyl chavicol which is contained in basil, therefore it is advisable to use with care.

BENZOIN

SUMMARY

Benzoin is a very useful oil for inflammatory skin conditions due to its soothing property, and for any condition in which fluid needs to be expelled from the body. It is also very valuable for general stress relief and nervous tension.

Botanical name: *Styrax benzoin*
Plant family: Styracaceae family
Aroma: sweet vanilla-like scent
Colour: orange, brown viscous oil
Method of production: by solvent extraction (the resin is collected from the bark of the tree by cutting triangular wounds into the bark, from which the

sap exudes). The crude benzoin is extracted from the trees directly, and benzoin resinoid or 'resin absolute' is prepared from the crude benzoin using solvents such as benzene and alcohol.

Main countries of production: Sumatra, Java and Malaysia for 'Sumatra' Benzoin and Vietnam, Cambodia, China and Thailand for 'Siam' Benzoin.

Therapeutic properties:

- antiseptic
- astringent
- anti-inflammatory
- vulnerary
- expectorant
- circulatory stimulant
- diuretic
- carminative
- nerve sedative.

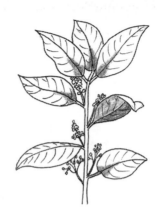

Figure 4
Benzoin

Therapeutic uses:

- poor circulation
- muscular aches and pains
- respiratory problems (bronchitis, asthma, coughs, sore throats)
- digestive problems (indigestion, flatulence)
- nervous exhaustion
- calms nervous tension
- skin care – healing to cracked, chapped skin
- cystitis.

Precautions:

- May cause sensitisation in some individuals.

BERGAMOT

SUMMARY

A very uplifting oil to both mind and body, invaluable for depression and stress-related conditions.

Botanical name: *Citrus bergamia*
Plant family: Rutaceae family
Aroma: light, delicate, refreshing and uplifting. It has a spicy lemon/orange scent with slight floral overtones.
Colour: greenish-brown colour
Method of extraction: expressed from the rind of a small, orange-like fruit
Main countries of production: Southern Italy, Sicily, Morocco

Therapeutic properties:

- antiseptic (pulmonary and genito-urinary)
- astringent
- antiviral
- febrifuge
- analgesic
- antispasmodic
- carminative
- laxative
- diuretic
- stomachic
- tonic
- rubefacient
- stimulant
- parasiticide
- vulnerary
- antidepressant
- uplifting.

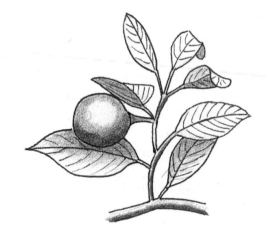

Figure 5
Bergamot

Therapeutic uses:

- respiratory problems
- digestive problems (dyspepsia, flatulence, colic, indigestion)
- urinary infections (cystitis)
- depression
- skin infections
- stress related conditions
- anxiety
- nervous tension
- depression and negativity
- skin care – acne, oily and congested skins.

Precautions:

- Bergamot contains certain chemical constituents called furocoumarins, notably *bergaptene*, which, upon exposure to strong sunlight, will increase the photosensitivity of the skin. Avoid direct contact with strong sunlight after using this oil, or substitute with the rectified version Bergamot FCF (furocoumarin free).

BLACK PEPPER

SUMMARY

Black pepper is very stimulating to mind and body and is particularly effective on the muscular and digestive systems.

Botanical name: *Piper Nigrum*
Plant family: Piperaceae family
Aroma: spicy, hot, very sharp aroma
Colour: colourless to pale greenish yellow.
Method of production: steam distilled from the crushed berries of the vine-like shrub. This oil is usually derived from black pepper, rather than white (hence its name) as black pepper is more aromatic and contains greater amounts of oil.
Main countries of production: cultivated in the East, mainly obtained from Singapore, India and Malaysia

Therapeutic properties:

- antiseptic
- antimicrobial
- analgesic
- rubefacient
- stimulant (circulatory, nervous and digestive)
- antispasmodic
- carminative
- laxative
- detoxicant
- febrifuge
- diuretic
- stomachic
- tonic.

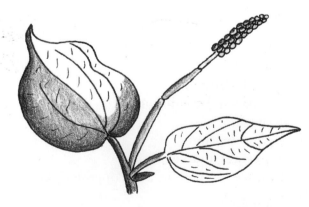

Figure 6
Black Pepper

Therapeutic uses:

- muscular aches and pains
- poor muscle tone
- poor circulation
- digestive problems (flatulence, colic, constipation, diarrhoea, loss of appetite, nausea)
- respiratory problems (colds, flu, viral infections).

Precautions:

- Use in low concentration as it may cause skin irritation.

ROMAN CHAMOMILE

SUMMARY

Best known for soothing and calming effects on the emotions as well as on many physical conditions, particularly those associated with the skin and the nervous and digestive systems.

Botanical name: *Anthemis nobilis*
Plant family: compositae family
Aroma: a fruity, apple-like fragrance
Colour: very pale greenish yellow
Method of extraction: steam distillation of the flower heads
Main countries of production: cultivated mainly in Britain, Belgium, France, Hungary, Italy and the USA

Therapeutic properties:

- antiseptic
- analgesic
- anti-inflammatory
- stimulant (increases white blood cell production)
- tonic
- calming
- soothing
- bactericidal
- antispasmodic
- carminative

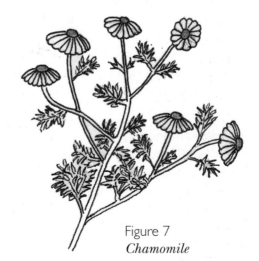

Figure 7
Chamomile

- stomachic
- antidepressant
- nerve sedative
- hypnotic
- vulnerary
- emmenagogue.

Therapeutic uses:

- muscular aches and pain (particularly dull aches)
- digestive problems (colic, dyspepsia, indigestion, nausea, diarrhoea)
- menstrual problems
- anaemia
- insomnia
- headaches
- migraine
- nervous tension
- anxiety
- nervous depression
- stress related disorders
- skin care – allergies, sensitive skins, inflammatory skin conditions.

Precautions:

- Avoid during the early months of pregnancy.
- Use in very low concentration as it may cause irritation.

GERMAN CHAMOMILE

SUMMARY

A very effective oil in skin care, particularly effective on allergies and inflammatory skin conditions. However, must be used with care to avoid adverse skin reaction.

Botanical name: *Matricaria chamomilia*
Plant family: compositae family
Aroma: German or blue chamomile has a herb-like, slightly sweet smell, but with a much 'heavier' note than Roman chamomile
Colour: deep blue, due to its high azulene content (azulene is not actually present in the plant, but is formed during the process of distillation)
Method of extraction: steam distillation of the flower heads

Main countries of production: German chamomile is cultivated mainly in Hungary and Eastern Europe and despite its name, is no longer grown in Germany

Therapeutic properties:

- analgesic
- anti-allergenic
- anti-inflammatory
- antispasmodic
- stomachic
- digestive
- analgesic
- bactericidal
- febrifuge
- fungicidal
- nerve sedative
- stimulant (of white blood cells)
- vulnerary
- emmenagogue.

Therapeutic uses:

- see Roman chamomile (page 38).

Precautions:

- Avoid during the early months of pregnancy.
- Use in very low concentration as it may cause sensitisation.

MOROCCAN CHAMOMILE

─── SUMMARY ───

Moroccan chamomile is different chemically and olfactorily to Roman and German chamomile and therefore does not share their extensive properties. It is generally quite soothing and calming on the nerves.

Botanical name: *Ormenis multicaulis*
Plant family: compositae family
Aroma: Moroccan chamomile has a fresh sweet herbaceous smell, which slightly resembles Roman chamomile
Colour: very pale greenish yellow

Method of extraction: steam distillation of the flower heads

Main countries of production: Moroccan chamomile is mainly cultivated in northwest Africa, Spain and Israel

Therapeutic properties:

- antispasmodic
- hepatic
- sedative
- emmenagogue.

Therapeutic uses:

- menstrual problems
- digestive problems
- insomnia
- headaches and migraine
- nervous irritability.

Precautions:

- Avoid during first part of pregnancy.

CLARY SAGE

SUMMARY

A deep muscle relaxant which is useful for helping the mind and body to relax simultaneously.

Botanical name: *Salvia sclarea*

Plant family: labiatae family

Aroma: heavy, herbal, nutty fragrance

Colour: pale yellow

Method of extraction: steam distilled from the fresh herb and flowering tops and foliage

Main countries of production: France, Morocco, Italy, Syria
Therapeutic properties:

- antispasmodic
- carminative
- muscle relaxant
- aphrodisiac
- euphoric
- antidepressant
- hypotensive
- emmenagogue
- regulates sebum
- nervine.

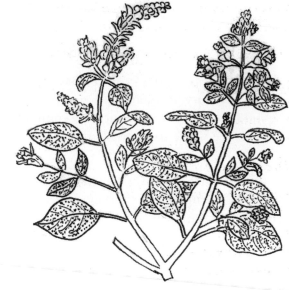

Figure 8
Clary Sage

Therapeutic uses:

- digestive problems (colic, dyspepsia, flatulence, intestinal cramps)
- respiratory problems (asthma, throat infections, bronchitis)
- menstrual cramps
- muscular aches and pains
- high blood pressure
- migraine
- nervous tension
- depression
- pre-menstrual syndrome
- skin care – acne, oily skin and hair.

Precautions:

- Avoid during pregnancy.
- Avoid combining the use of clary sage with alcohol as it may cause drowsiness.

CYPRESS

━━ S U M M A R Y ━━

The key property of cypress is that it is a powerful astringent, excellent for circulatory problems and an effective 'hormonal' oil. Reputedly good for coughs and respiratory complaints (in France, cough pastilles were once made from crushed cypress cones).

Botanical name: *Cupressus sempervirens*
Plant family: cupresaceae family
Aroma: a pleasant smoky, woody smell, yet is clear and refreshing
Colour: colourless or a very pale yellow
Method of extraction: steam distilled from the needles, twigs and cones of the tree
Main countries of production: The tree is native to eastern Mediterranean. Most of the oil comes from trees cultivated in France, Spain and Morocco.

Therapeutic properties:

- antiseptic
- astringent
- antispasmodic
- anti-rheumatic
- deodorant
- diuretic
- hepatic
- tonic
- vasoconstrictive
- regulates the menstrual cycle.

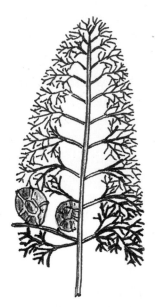

Figure 9
Cypress

Therapeutic uses:

- respiratory problems (asthma, whooping cough, bronchitis)
- menstrual problems (excessive bleeding)
- menopausal symptoms

- poor circulation
- oedema
- varicose veins
- haemorrhoids
- excessive perspiration
- muscular aches and pains (rheumatism)
- skin care – acne, oily skin and hair
- nervous tension
- irritability.

Precautions:

- There are no specific precautions associated with cypress, as it is generally considered to be non-toxic, non-irritant and non-sensitising.

EUCALYPTUS (BLUE GUM)

— SUMMARY —

A very powerful oil, having powerful effects on the respiratory system, and an excellent agent in healing flesh wounds and external ulcers.

Botanical name: *Eucalyptus Globulus*
Plant family: myrtaceae family
Aroma: clear, sharp, penetrating and piercing; camphoraceous with a woody-scent undertone, is head-clearing and cooling
Colour: colourless liquid (pale yellow on ageing)
Method of extraction: steam distilled from the fresh or partially dried leaves and young twigs
Main countries of production: native to Australia and Tasmania. Mainly cultivated in Spain, Portugal, Brazil, California, Russia and China.

Therapeutic properties:

- antibiotic
- antiviral
- decongestant
- expectorant
- febrifuge
- antiseptic
- bactericidal
- vulnerary
- anti-rheumatic
- rubefacient
- analgesic
- stimulant
- depurative
- diuretic.

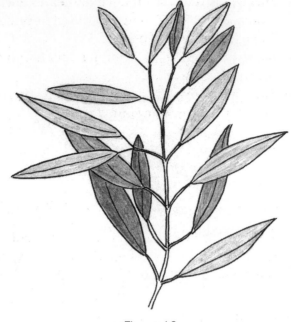

Figure 10
Eucalyptus

Therapeutic uses:

- respiratory problems (coughs, head colds, asthma, bronchitis, flu, catarrh, sinusitis)
- muscular aches and pains
- poor circulation
- cystitis
- debility
- skin care – healing to cuts, wounds, ulcers, burns and blisters, skin infections.

Precautions:

- Eucalyptus oil is a powerful oil and therefore should be used in low concentrations.
- May antidote homeopathic medication due to its strong odour.
- Although externally non-toxic, non-irritant (in dilution) and non-sensitising, when taken internally eucalyptus is toxic and as little as 3.5 ml has been reported as fatal.

Additional note

There are approximately 500 species of eucalyptus which produce a type of essential oil:

- **Eucalyptus Radiata**   the narrow-leaves eucalyptus with a sweeter, less harsh aroma. This type is sometimes used in preference to the blue gum type, due to its sweeter odour.
- **Eucalyptus Citiadora**   lemon scented with a strong, fresh citronella-like aroma.
- **Eucalyptus Dives**   broad leaved peppermint which has a fresh, camphoraceous, spicy-minty aroma.

FENNEL

———— SUMMARY ————

Well known for its tonic action on digestion and for its detoxifying character (Fennel has long been an ingredient of baby gripe water, along with its fellow unbellifer, dill).

Botanical name: *Foeniculum vulgare*
Plant family: umbelliferae family
Aroma: very characteristic smell of aniseed, both floral and herby, is slightly spicy
Colour: usually colourless, sometimes a very pale yellow
Method of extraction: steam distilled from the crushed seeds of the herb
Main countries of production: native to the Mediterranean. Most of the oil is produced in Eastern Europe, Germany, France, Italy and Greece.

Therapeutic properties:

- anti-inflammatory
- aperitif
- antimicrobial
- antiseptic
- antispasmodic
- carminative
- depurative
- detoxicant
- diuretic
- emmenagogue
- laxative
- circulatory stimulant
- stomachic
- tonic.

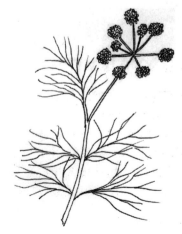

Figure 11
Fennel

Therapeutic uses:

- digestive problems (colic, constipation, dyspepsia, flatulence, nausea)
- urinary tract infections
- respiratory problems (asthma, bronchitis)
- menstrual problems
- menopausal problems
- poor circulation
- cellulite
- skin care – dull, oily and mature skins, helps reduce bruising, tightens and tones skin.

Precautions:

- Fennel is a very powerful oil, therefore use in moderation.
- It is best avoided during pregnancy.
- It is best avoided by sufferers of epilepsy.
- Take care when blending, as one drop too many may overkill the blend.
- Only ever use sweet fennel and NOT bitter fennel in aromatherapy.

FRANKINCENSE

Note: also known as **Olibanum**

——— S U M M A R Y ———

The chief uses of frankincense are in skin care and respiratory infections.

Botanical name: *Botswellia carteri*
Plant family: burseraceae family
Aroma: a woody, warm spicy fragrance, with a subtle hint of lemon
Colour: colourless or pale yellow
Method of extraction: steam distilled from the resin of the bark of the tree by steam distillation
Main countries of production: North and East Africa, Arab countries, Middle East, China. Although the raw material is mainly produced in Somalia and Ethiopia, most of the oil is distilled in Europe.

Therapeutic properties:

- antiseptic
- expectorant
- uterine
- affinity for urino-genital tract
- astringent
- cytophylactic
- anti-inflammatory
- sedative
- calming
- emmenagogue.

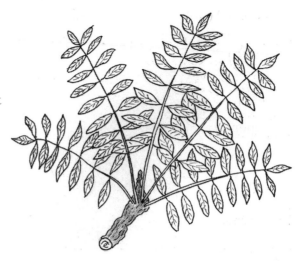

Figure 12
Frankincense

Therapeutic uses:

- respiratory problems (asthma, bronchitis, coughs, colds, laryngitis and catarrhal conditions)
- menstrual problems
- urinary and genital infections
- depression
- nervous tension
- skin care – mature skins, effective on acne, abscesses, scars, blemishes and wounds.

Precautions:

- Best avoided during the first part of pregnancy.

GERANIUM

SUMMARY

A balancing and regulating oil which tends to balance extremes, whether on the physical or emotional level.

Botanical name: *Pelargonium graveolens*
Plant family: geraniaceae family
Aroma: sweet and heavy, rather like rose, but with minty overtones

Colour: fairly colourless with a faint tinge of green
Method of extraction: steam distillation from the aromatic green parts of the pelargonium, especially the leaves
Main countries of production: France, Reunion, Spain, Morocco, Egypt and Italy

Therapeutic properties:

- antiseptic
- astringent
- anti-inflammatory
- antihaemorrhagic
- antidepressant
- homeostatic
- stimulant of the adrenal cortex
- diuretic
- tonic (to liver and kidneys)
- vulnerary.

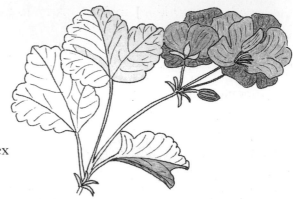

Figure 13
Geranium

Therapeutic uses:

- hormone imbalances (premenstrual syndrome, menopausal problems)
- cellulite
- poor circulation
- fluid retention
- oedema
- anxiety and depression
- skin care – effective on skin types, especially dry and oily.

Precautions:

- May cause some irritation to sensitive skins.
- May cause restlessness if used excessively.

GINGER

SUMMARY

A very warming oil, which has very positive effects on the muscular, digestive and nervous systems.

Botanical name: *Zingiber officinale*
Plant family: zingiberaceae family
Aroma: warm woody-spicy scent
Colour: pale yellow, amber liquid
Method of extraction: steam distilled from the dried ground root
Main countries of production: native to Southern Asia and is cultivated across the West Indies, China, Jamaica, Japan. Most of the oil is distilled in China, India and Britain.

Main therapeutic properties:

- analgesic
- antiseptic
- aphrodisiac
- bactericidal
- antispasmodic
- carminative
- stomachic
- expectorant
- febrifuge
- laxative
- rubefacient
- stimulant
- tonic.

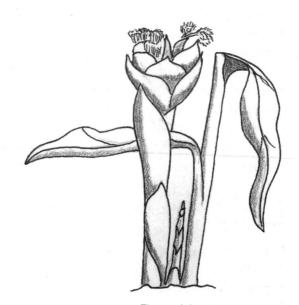

Figure 14
Ginger

Main therapeutic uses:

- muscular aches and pains
- poor circulation
- respiratory problems (coughs, colds, sore throats, flu)
- digestive problems (diarrhoea, indigestion, colic, loss of appetite, nausea)
- nervous exhaustion.

Precautions:

- May cause irritation to sensitive skin, therefore use in low concentration.

GRAPEFRUIT

SUMMARY

A very effective oil for stimulating the lymphatic system. It is uplifting, and will help depression and general stress-related conditions.

Botanical name: *Citrus paradisi*
Plant family: rutaceae family
Aroma: fresh, sweet, sharp and refreshing citrus aroma
Colour: virtually colourless, very pale yellow or green
Method of extraction: cold expressed from the fresh peel of the fruit
Main countries of production: native to Asia and the West Indies. The oil is mainly produced in California, Florida, Brazil and Israel.

Therapeutic properties:

- antiseptic
- antitoxic
- astringent
- bactericidal
- stimulant (lymphatic and digestive)
- diuretic
- depurative
- tonic
- calming and slightly hypnotic.

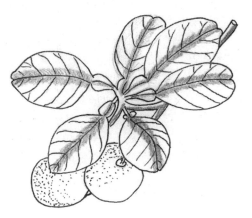

Figure 15
Grapefruit

Therapeutic uses:

- respiratory problems (coughs, colds, flu)
- cellulite
- fluid retention
- muscle fatigue
- nervous exhaustion
- depression
- headaches
- skin care (acne, congested and oily skins).

Precautions:

- Unlike other citrus oils, grapefruit is not phototoxic.
- It has a relatively short shelf life and will oxidise quickly. Once oxidised, it will cause skin irritation and sensitisation.

JASMINE

—— **SUMMARY** ——

At any time, jasmine makes a luxurious and extremely enjoyable massage oil. Culpeper in his herbal said "The oil is good for hard and contracted limbs, it opens, warms and softens the nerves and tendons . . ."

Most notably used for its effects on the reproductive system, the skin and as an effective oil for depression.

Botanical name: *Jasminum officinale*
Plant family: oleaceae family
Aroma: very sweet, flowery, heavy and supremely exotic. Slightly heady, warming and intoxicating
Colour: the absolute is dark orange-brown and very viscous
Method of extraction: solvent extraction of the flowers. The jasmine flower increases in odour after dark due to the actual changes in the internal chemistry of the flower at night, and so harvesting the flowers has to be done at night to obtain a good quality oil, with consequent increases in labour costs.
Main countries of production: S. France, Tunisia, Morocco, Egypt, China and India (Egyptian and French jasmine is said to be the most superior quality).

Therapeutic properties:

- antiseptic
- mild analgesic
- antidepressant
- anti-inflammatory
- expectorant
- aphrodisiac
- uterine tonic
- antispasmodic
- parturient.

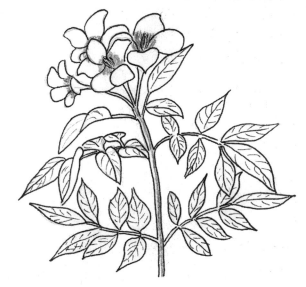

Figure 16
Jasmine

Therapeutic uses:

- muscular aches and pains, stiff limbs
- respiratory problems (coughs, colds, laryngitis)
- menstrual pain
- labour pain
- reproductive problems
- depression and confidence boosting
- skin care – effective on all skin types especially the hot, dry and sensitive skins. Also effective on scarring.

Precautions:

- Jasmine should not be used in pregnancy until the expectant mother is about to give birth, when it can be used to help labour.
- The powerful aroma indicates that this oil should be used in low proportions only.
- Due to the high cost of production, jasmine is often adulterated.

JUNIPER BERRY

—— S U M M A R Y ——

A thoroughly 'cleansing' oil which works effectively on an emotional and physical plane.

Botanical name: *Juniperus communis*
Plant family: cupressaceae family
Aroma: clear, refreshing, slightly woody, quite similar to pine
Colour: transparent, colourless, sometimes with a slight tinge of greenish yellow
Method of extraction: distilled from the fresh black ripe berries of the bush/evergreen shrub
Main countries of production: Hungary, France, Italy, Yugoslavia, Canada. Those from Italy and France are reputed to be of the better quality.

Therapeutic properties:

- antiseptic
- astringent
- anti-rheumatic

- rubefacient
- depurative
- nervine
- sedative
- diuretic
- detoxifying
- stimulant
- antispasmodic
- stomachic
- tonic
- emmenagogue
- vulnerary.

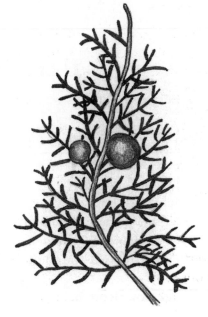

Figure 17
Juniper berry

Therapeutic uses:

- muscular aches and pains; stiff limbs
- poor circulation
- fluid retention
- cystitis
- accumulation of toxic waste
- anxiety and nervous tension
- menstrual problems
- skin care – effective for acne, congested and oily skins. Also effective for weepy eczema, psoriasis and dermatitis.

Precautions:

- Best avoided during pregnancy.
- Use in moderation as it can be very stimulating.
- Do not use juniper in the case of severe kidney disorders.

LAVENDER

── **S U M M A R Y** ──

Lavender is best known for its versatility, being effective on a wide range of conditions.

Botanical name: *Lavendula Officinalis*
Plant family: labiatae family
Aroma: light, clear and floral with woody undertones, very highly scented. The French lavender is considered better than the English, because it is richer in linalyl acetate which gives it a fruitier and sweeter note, whereas the English lavender has a more camphoric smell, with higher proportions of lineol.
Colour: varies in colour from being virtually colourless to dark yellow or dark greeny-yellow
Method of extraction: steam distillation from the fresh flowering tops of the plant
Main countries of production: England, France and Mediterranean countries.

Therapeutic properties:

- antiseptic
- analgesic
- cytophylactic
- antibiotic
- antiviral
- bactericidal
- decongestant
- antispasmodic
- carminative
- hypotensive
- rubefacient
- anti-rheumatic
- sedative
- antidepressant
- calming
- soothing
- vulnerary

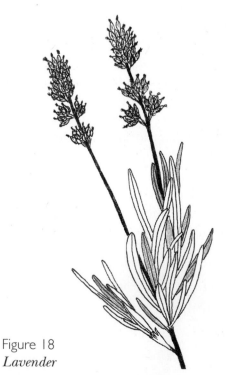

Figure 18
Lavender

- diuretic
- nervine
- insecticidal
- emmenagogue.

Therapeutic uses:

- muscular aches and pains
- respiratory problems (colds, coughs, sinusitis, flu, asthma and bronchitis)
- digestive problems (colic, dyspepsia, flatulence and nausea)
- high blood pressure
- painful menstruation
- labour pain
- headaches
- depression
- skin care – promotes rapid healing, effective for most skin types.

Precautions:

- Best avoided during first part of pregnancy.

LEMON

———— SUMMARY ————

Lemon is a refreshing and cooling oil and its key function is strengthening the immune system.

Botanical name: *Citrus limonum*
Plant family: rutaceae family
Aroma: sharp and fresh, citrussy smell
Colour: pale yellow, sometimes with a green tinge
Method of extraction: expressed from the oily rind of the fruit
Main countries of production: Sicily, Italy, Spain, Portugal, California, S. France.

Therapeutic properties:

- antiseptic
- astringent
- anti-anaemic
- anti-rheumatic

- antispasmodic
- carminative
- bactericidal
- depurative
- febrifuge
- homeostatic
- hypotensive
- insecticidal
- rubefacient
- stimulates white blood cells
- tonic.

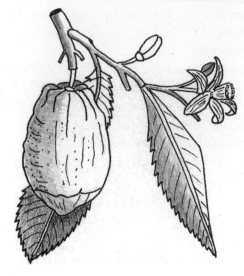

Figure 19
Lemon

Therapeutic uses:

- poor circulation
- high blood pressure
- respiratory problems (sore throats, colds, flu, bronchitis)
- digestive problems (indigestion, gastric acidity, bloatedness)
- skin care – oily skin, cuts and wounds.

Precautions:

- As lemon is a fairly strong astringent, it may cause skin irritation and sensitisation, therefore use in moderation.
- Lemon is phototoxic, therefore do not use on skin exposed directly to strong sunlight.

LEMONGRASS

━━━━ SUMMARY ━━━━

A very powerful antiseptic, useful in combating infection and a valuable stress-relieving oil, with a pleasant fresh smell.

Botanical name: *Cymbopogon citratus/flexuosus*
Plant family: gramineae family
Aroma: very sweet and lemony, like the smell of sherbert lemons, a fresh

grassy scent. The East Indian type has a slightly lighter fragrance.
Colour: West Indian lemongrass is reddish amber and the East Indian type is yellowish
Method of extraction: steam distilled from the fresh and partially dried grass
Main countries of production: Originally from India, it also grows in other tropical areas such as Brazil, the West and East Indies, Sri Lanka and China.

Therapeutic properties:

- antiseptic
- astringent
- analgesic
- antidepressant
- bactericidal
- carminative
- deodorant
- febrifuge
- nervine
- nerve sedative
- tonic.

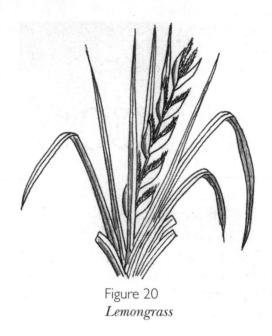

Figure 20
Lemongrass

Therapeutic uses:

- tired aching muscles
- digestive problems (colitis, indigestion, flatulence)
- respiratory problems (sore throats and fevers)
- excessive perspiration
- fatigue (mental and physical)
- nervous exhaustion
- headaches
- stress related conditions
- skin care – acne, infectious skin conditions, especially effective on open pores and oily skins.

Precautions:

- This oil has the potential to cause dermal irritation/sensitisation in some individuals and therefore a low dilution is recommended.
- This oil is sometimes used to assist the adulteration of more costly oils such as Melissa.

MARJORAM (SWEET)

——— S U M M A R Y ———

Marjoram is a powerful muscle relaxant, which allows the mind and body to relax simultaneously. It has a particularly soothing, warming and fortifying effect on disorders of the digestive, muscular, nervous and respiratory systems.

Botanical name: *Origanum marjorana*
Plant family: labiatae family
Aroma: slightly spicy, warming and penetrating, has a peppery, nutty and slightly camphorish note
Colour: pale to greenish yellow, becoming darker when older
Method of production: steam distillation from the dried leaves/flowering tops of the herb
Main countries of production: Sweet marjoram originates from Libya, Egypt and the Mediterranean, although much is obtained from France.

Therapeutic properties:

- analgesic
- rubefacient
- heart sedative
- arterial vasodilator
- hypotensive
- antispasmodic
- carminative
- laxative
- antiseptic
- antiviral
- expectorant
- nervine
- anaphrodisiac
- emmenagogue.

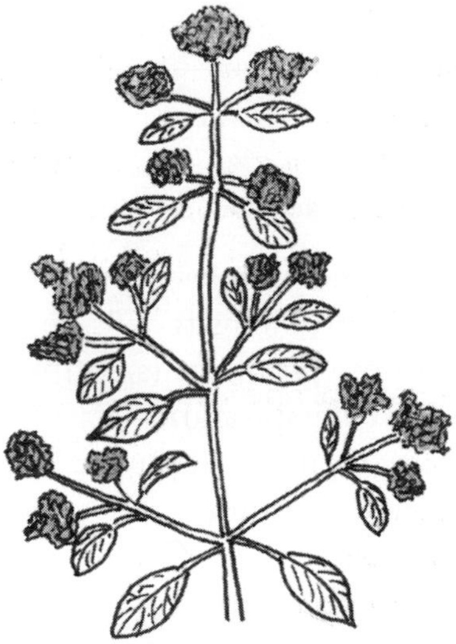

Figure 21
Marjoram (sweet)

Therapeutic uses:

- tight, painful muscles, overexertion
- musculo-skeletal problems – arthritis, rheumatism
- high blood pressure and heart conditions
- migraine

- digestive problems (indigestion, constipation, flatulence)
- menstrual pain
- respiratory problems (colds, coughs, bronchitis, asthma)
- insomnia
- nervous tension
- stress-related disorders.

Precautions:

- The use of marjoram is best avoided during pregnancy.

NEROLI (ORANGE BLOSSOM)

SUMMARY

Neroli is a wonderfully effective oil for stress relief and is the best oil for shock.

Botanical name: *Citrus aurantium var. amara*
Plant family: rutacea family
Aroma: very sweet and floral with a bitter undertone
Colour: pale yellow liquid (absolute is a dark brown or orange viscous liquid)
Method of extraction: steam distilled from the freshly picked blooms
Main countries of production: native to the Far East but cultivated extensively in the Mediterranean region. Major producers include Italy, Tunisia, Morocco, Egypt and France.

Therapeutic properties:

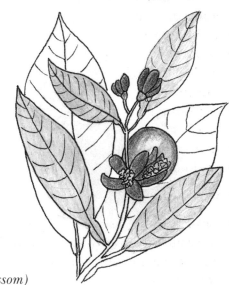

- antiseptic
- bactericidal
- cytophylactic
- antispasmodic
- carminative
- circulatory and cardiac tonic
- nervine
- antidepressant
- mildly hypnotic.

Figure 22
Neroli (orange blossom)

Therapeutic uses:

- skin care (all skin types especially dry, sensitive and mature), also effective for stretch marks and scar tissue
- poor circulation
- palpitations
- digestive problems (especially those which are stress-related)
- depression
- nervous tension
- anxiety and stress related disorders.

Precautions:

- Neroli has no known hazards.

ORANGE (SWEET)

SUMMARY

Orange is very 'cheery' and can help to dispel nervous tension whether purely emotional or linked to a physical ailment.

Botanical name: *Citrus Aurantium Sinensis*
Plant family: rutaceae family
Aroma: vivid sweet orange-fruity aroma, the bitter oil has a slightly more delicate smell than the sweet. Has a warm and penetrating smell, zesty
Colour: deep golden yellow
Method of production: expressed from the outer, coloured part of the rind
Main countries of production: W. Indies, China, Israel.

Therapeutic properties:

- antiseptic
- bactericidal
- antispasmodic
- carminative
- hypotensive
- stomachic
- tonic
- stimulant (digestive and lymphatic)
- mild nerve sedative
- antidepressant.

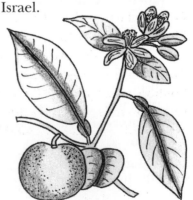

Figure 23
Orange (sweet)

Therapeutic uses:

- respiratory problems (colds and flu)
- digestive problems (indigestion, constipation, diarrhoea, irritable bowel syndrome)
- nervous tension
- anxiety and depression
- insomnia
- skin care – good skin tonic, effective on congested and dry skins.

Precautions:

- The distilled oil is phototoxic and although the expressed oil contains coumarins, there is no evidence to suggest that *it* is phototoxic. The oil extracted from the bitter orange is far more likely to cause phototoxicity, nevertheless caution is advised.

PATCHOULI

--- **S U M M A R Y** ---

Patchouli is very useful in skin care, being a very effective cell regenerator. Dried patchouli leaves were placed amongst the folds of India cashmere shawls in Victorian times to protect the merchandise from moths. Patchouli was much 'in vogue' during the Flower Power of the 1960's.

Unlike other essences, patchouli seems to improve with age.

Botanical name: *Pogostemon cablin*
Plant family: labiatae family
Aroma: sweet rich earthy odour, is strong and exotic, slightly spicy
Colour: amber, dark orange viscous oil
Method of extraction: steam distillation of the dried leaves
Main countries of production: native to Asia, Indonesia and the Philippines, also grown in India, China, Malaysia and South America.

Therapeutic properties:

- antiseptic
- antiviral
- astringent
- antimicrobial
- cytophylactic
- anti-inflammatory
- febrifuge
- fungicidal
- deodorant
- diuretic
- nervine
- sedative
- tonic
- antidepressant
- aphrodisiac.

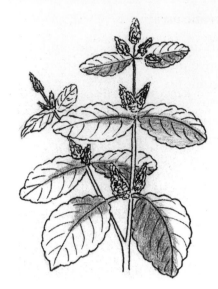

Figure 24
Patchouli

Therapeutic uses:

- poor circulation
- fluid retention
- muscular aches and pains
- depression
- nervous exhaustion
- stress-related conditions
- excessive perspiration
- skin care – oily skin and hair, effective on skin infections (fungal and bacterial), healing to cracked skin.

Precautions:

- Generally regarded as non-irritant and non-sensitising.
- As patchouli is highly odoriferous, use sparingly.

PEPPERMINT

SUMMARY

A very stimulating oil to both mind and body, particularly known for its effects on digestion and the respiratory system.

Botanical name: *Mentha piperita*
Plant family: labiatae family
Aroma: strong, sharp, fresh piercing menthol fragrance
Colour: colourless or very pale yellow
Method of production: steam distillation from the herb/whole plant
Main countries of production: England, USA.

Therapeutic properties:

- antiseptic
- antiviral
- decongestant
- expectorant
- febrifuge
- antispasmodic
- carminative
- analgesic
- anti-inflammatory
- cephalic
- nervine.

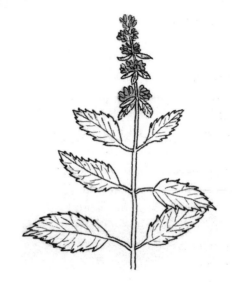

Figure 25
Peppermint

Therapeutic uses:

- digestive upsets (nausea, colic, cramp, dyspepsia, flatulence)
- respiratory problems (asthma, bronchitis, sinusitis, colds, flu)
- feverish conditions
- headaches
- fatigue (mental and physical)
- skin care – congested skin conditions
- shock.

Precautions

- As peppermint is very stimulating, use in moderation.
- May cause sensitisation in some individual due to menthol constituent.
- Best avoided during first part of pregnancy.
- Avoid this oil if homeopathic remedies are being taken, as it may antidote them.

PETITGRAIN

─── **SUMMARY** ───

Petitgrain has very beneficial effects on digestive and minor stress-related conditions and is very refreshing.

Botanical name: *Citrus aurantium var. amara*
Plant family: rutaceae family
Aroma: fresh, invigorating, slightly floral citrus scent with a woody-herbaceous undertone. Resembles neroli but with a less bitter note
Colour: pale yellow to amber liquid
Method of production: steam distilled from the leaves and twigs of the same tree that produces bitter orange oil and orange blossom oil (neroli)
Main countries of production: native of China and N. and E. India. The best quality oil is said to come from France but good quality oils are also produced in N. Africa, Italy, Egypt, Tunisia, Paraguay and Haiti.

Therapeutic properties:

- antiseptic
- antidepressant
- antispasmodic
- deodorant
- digestive
- nervine
- stomachic
- tonic
- antidepressant.

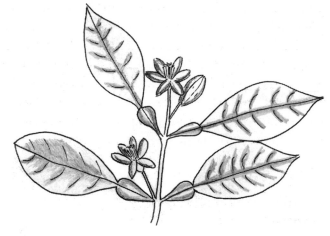

Figure 26
Petitgrain

Therapeutic uses:

- excessive perspiration
- digestive problems (dyspepsia, flatulence, indigestion)
- insomnia
- nervous exhaustion
- stress related conditions
- skin care – acne and oily skins.

Precautions

- Petitgrain has no known hazards.

ROSE

——— SUMMARY ———

Rose is a superb oil; it is effective for skin care, and has an affinity with the female reproductive system. Rose also has a pronounced effect on the circulation, digestion and nervous systems.

Botanical name: *Rosa dameascena* (damask rose is also known as *rose otto*) and *rosa centifolia* (cabbage rose or rose absolute)

Plant family: rosaceae family

Aroma: the damask rose or rose otto has a sweet and mellow scent with a hint of cloves and vanilla. The cabbage rose or rose absolute has a deep rich sweet honey-rose aroma

Colour: rose otto is virtually colourless liquid which becomes semi-solid at room temperature, and rose absolute is a yellowy-orange viscous liquid

Method of extraction: rose otto is produced by steam distillation of the fresh petals and rose absolute is obtained by solvent extraction of the fresh petals

Main countries of production: the cabbage rose is mainly produced in Morocco, Tunisia, Italy, France and China. The best damask rose, known as rose otto comes from Bulgaria, although excellent varieties are also produced in Turkey and France.

Therapeutic properties:

- antidepressant
- anti-inflammatory
- antiseptic
- antispasmodic
- stomachic
- sedative
- haemostatic
- antiviral
- astringent
- tonic
- uterine
- emmenagogue.

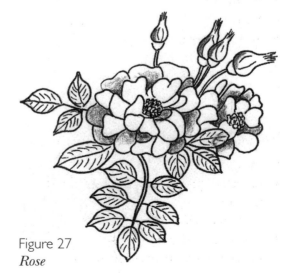

Figure 27
Rose

Therapeutic uses:

- menstrual problems (irregular or excessive)
- hormonal problems (premenstrual syndrome and menopause)
- depression
- nervous tension
- poor circulation
- emotional trauma
- skin care – all skin types especially for the dry, ageing and sensitive skins.

Precautions:

- Rose is generally considered to be non-toxic, non-irritant and non-sensitising.
- Because of the price of rose oil, it is often falsified and adulterated, with synthetic substitutes being widely used.

ROSEMARY

——— SUMMARY ———

A physical and mental stimulant, useful for a wide range of nervous, circulatory, muscular and digestive complaints.

Botanical name: *Rosemarinus officinalis*
Plant family: labiatae family
Aroma: a strong, herbal fragrance with a clear, warming and penetrating note. The poorer quality oils have a strong camphorous smell
Colour: virtually colourless or slightly pale yellow green
Method of production: steam distillation from the flower/leaves of the herb
Main countries of production: France, Tunisia and Spain.

Therapeutic properties:

- analgesic
- antiseptic
- astringent
- antispasmodic
- anti-rheumatic
- hypertensive
- cephalic
- diuretic
- emmenagogue
- antispasmodic
- rubefacient
- aphrodisiac
- nervine
- stimulant of the central nervous system.

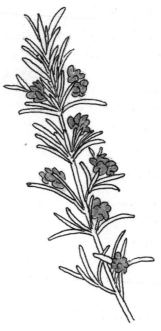

Figure 28
Rosemary

Therapeutic uses:

- muscular aches and pains
- respiratory problems (colds, catarrh, bronchitis, sinusitis, asthma)
- poor circulation
- cellulite
- fluid retention
- menstrual pain
- headaches and migraine
- fatigue (mental and physical)
- nervous exhaustion
- skin care – especially effective on oily skin and scalp disorders.

Precautions:

- Due to its highly stimulating actions, rosemary is not suitable for sufferers of epilepsy and those who suffer from hypertension.
- Best avoided in pregnancy.
- It is thought that, due to its piercing quality, rosemary may antidote homeopathic remedies.

SANDALWOOD

SUMMARY

A very subtle oil but with powerful effects on the skin and the respiratory system. Also a valuable antidepressant and aid to stress conditions, especially when associated with anxiety.

Botanical name: *Santalum album*

Plant family: santalaceae family

Aroma: woody and exotic, very subtle but is lingering and persistent. Is a very viscous oil

Colour: develops from a very pale yellow to a brownish yellow

Method of production: distilled from the heartwood of the Sandalwood tree (santalum album) after the outer wood has been eaten away by ants

Main countries of production: the best Sandalwood (santalum album) comes from the province of Mysore, India and grows from various islands of the Indian Ocean. Santalum spicatum, the Australian Sandalwood, is reputed to yield an inferior oil.

Therapeutic properties:

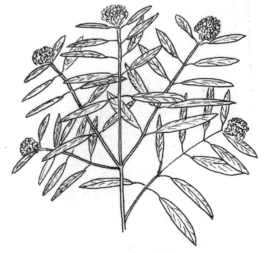

- antiseptic (pulmonary and urinar
- astringent
- bactericidal
- antispasmodic
- carminative
- diuretic
- expectorant
- aphrodisiac
- antidepressant
- sedative
- tonic.

Figure 29
Sandalwood

Therapeutic uses:

- respiratory problems (sore throats, chest infections, dry coughs, bronchitis, laryngitis)
- digestive problems (diarrhoea, nausea)
- cellulite

- cystitis
- insomnia
- depression
- nervous tension and anxiety
- skin care – effective on dry, dehydrated, oily skins and acne.

Precautions:

- Generally considered as non-toxic, non-irritant and non-sensitising.
- Lower concentrations of this oil are very effective and though the odour is not very pronounced when in the bottle, is very powerful when applied to the skin and also very persistent.

TEATREE

SUMMARY

The effects of teatree are diverse in that it is a very effective antiseptic in skin care and with respiratory ailments. Its key quality is in strengthening the immune system.

Botanical name: *Malaleuca alternifolia*
Plant family: myrtaceae family
Aroma: strong antiseptic, slightly milder than eucalyptus with a slight camphorish smell
Colour: usually yellowy green, but can be whiteish
Method of production: steam distilled from the leaves and twigs of the small tree or shrub
Main countries of production: native to Australia, New South Wales.

Therapeutic properties:

- antiseptic
- antibiotic
- antiviral
- antibacterial
- expectorant
- immune stimulant
- anti-inflammatory
- vulnerary
- parasiticidal
- fungicidal.

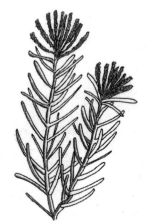

Figure 30
Teatree

Therapeutic uses:

- respiratory problems (asthma, bronchitis, coughs, colds, sinusitis)
- urinary infections (thrush and cystitis)
- building immunity against infection
- skin care – skin infections, infected wounds, burns, cold sores, spots.

Precautions

- Teatree may cause irritation and sensitisation to some skins.

THYME (SWEET)

SUMMARY

A very strong antiseptic, very effective on the pulmonary and genito-urinary systems.

Botanical name: *Thymus Vulgaris*
Plant family: labiatae family
Aroma: sweet herbaceous, warming aroma
Colour: pale yellow liquid
Method of extraction: steam distilled from the flowering tops/leaves of the herb
Main countries of production: mainly produced in Spain, but is also produced in France, Israel, Greece, Morocco, Algeria, Germany and the USA.

Therapeutic properties:

- antiseptic
- antiviral
- antibiotic
- antimicrobial
- anti-rheumatic
- expectorant
- antispasmodic
- carminative
- circulatory stimulant
- immune stimulant
- diuretic
- nervine
- rubefacient

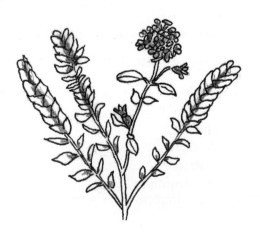

Figure 31
Thyme (sweet)

- hypertensive
- parasiticidal
- insecticidal
- emmenagogue.

Therapeutic uses:

- digestive problems (diarrhoea, dyspepsia, flatulence, intestinal cramp)
- respiratory problems (colds, sore throats, coughs, laryngitis, pharyngitis, whooping cough, asthma, bronchitis)
- muscular aches and pains
- poor circulation
- cystitis
- accumulation of toxins
- building immunity; infectious illnesses
- fatigue (mental and physical)
- nervous exhaustion
- skin care – abscesses, boils, cuts and skin infections.

Precautions

- Thyme is one of the strongest antiseptics and therefore should be used with care and in moderation.
- Avoid using thyme during pregnancy or in cases of high blood pressure.
- There are a number of chemotypes of thyme available but only a few are actually recommended for therapeutic use. Red thyme for example contains large amounts of toxic chemical constituents phenols which may cause skin irritation and sensitisation.
- White thyme is not a 'complete' oil; it is a redistillate of red thyme and is often adulterated.
- The oil labelled as 'sweet thyme' is preferable in aromatherapy as it contains higher amounts of more gentle constituents alcohols such as geraniol and linalol.
- Thyme citiadora, another species of thyme has a fresh scent and is less toxic than red or white thyme; it is therefore safe for use on the skin and on children.

YLANG YLANG

———— SUMMARY ————

A real 'comforter' in terms of treating stress as it is a very valuable anti-depressant and can help to instil confidence.

Botanical name: *Cananga odorata*

Plant family: anonaceae family

Aroma: sweet, floral but very heavy; a rather 'exotic' smell

Colour: colourless to a pale yellow

Method of production: distillation of the fresh flowers of the small tropical tree (the finer oil is distilled from the yellow blossoms, although there are pink and mauve varieties). The first distillate which is drawn off during the steam distillation process is of the highest quality and is sold under the name of 'Ylang Ylang'; the 'tail' part of the distillate is of a poorer grade and is sold under the name of 'Cananga'.

Main countries of production: Seychelles, Mauritius, Tahiti; the best oil is reputed to come from the Philippines.

Therapeutic properties:

- antiseptic
- aphrodisiac
- hypotensor
- nerve sedative
- nervine
- hypotensive
- circulatory stimulant
- tonic
- regulates sebum
- hormone regulator
- antidepressant
- euphoric
- uterine tonic.

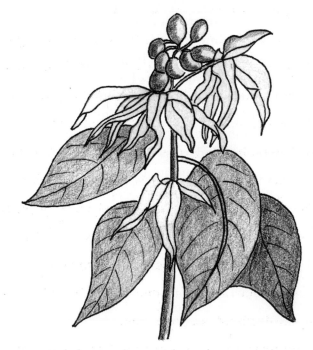

Figure 32
Ylang Ylang

Therapeutic uses:

- nervous tension
- anxiety
- panic attacks
- high blood pressure
- insomnia
- hormonal problems
- skin care – oily and dry skins, tonic to the scalp.

Precautions:

- May cause sensitisation in some skins.
- Due to its rather sickly sweet smell, using it in excessive quantities can lead to headaches and nausea, both for the client and the therapist.

GLOSSARY OF THERAPEUTIC PROPERTIES

Analgesic: relieves pain

Anaphrodisiac: reduces sexual desire

Anti-anaemic: an agent which helps combat anaemia

Antibiotic: prevents the growth of, or destroys, bacteria

Antidepressant: uplifting, counteracting melancholy, alleviates depression

Anti-inflammatory: alleviates inflammation

Anti-microbial: destroys or resists pathogenic micro-organisms

Anti-rheumatic: helps relieve and prevent rheumatism

Antiseptic: destroys and prevents the development of microbes

Antispasmodic: relieves cramp, prevents or eases spasms or convulsions

Antiviral: substance which inhibits the growth of a virus

Anti-haemorrhagic: prevents or combats bleeding

Aperitif: stimulates the appetite

Aphrodisiac: increases or stimulates sexual desire

Astringent: contracts bodily tissues, helps to control infection

Bactericidal: an agent that destroys bacteria

Carminative: relieves flatulence (wind) by expelling gas from the intestines

Cephalic: stimulates and clears the mind

Cytophylactic: encourages cell regeneration

Decongestant: releases nasal mucous

Deodorant: reduces odour

Depurative: helps combat impurities, detoxifying

Detoxifying/detoxicant: helps cleanse the body of impurities

Diuretic: stimulates the secretion of urine

Emmenagogue: induces or assists menstruation

Expectorant: aids removal of catarrh

Febrifuge: combats fever

Fungicidal: kills or inhibits the growth of yeasts, moulds etc.

Homeostatic: arrests bleeding/haemorrhage

Hepatic: tonic to the liver, aids functioning of liver

Hypertensive: increases blood pressure

Hypotensive: lowers blood pressure

Hormonal: balances or regulates the body's hormonal secretion

Immunostimulant: stimulates the body's own natural defence system

Insecticidal: repels insects

Laxative: promotes elimination of the bowels

Nervine: strengthens the nervous system

Parasiticidal: destroys and prevents parasites

Parturient: aids childbirth

Relaxant: soothes, induces relaxation, relieves strain or tension

Rubefacient: increases local circulation, creates erythema, warming

Sedative: produces a calming effect

Stimulant: has a rousing, uplifting effect on the mind and body

Stomachic: digestive aid and tonic, improves appetite

Tonic: strengthens and enlivens the whole or specific parts of the body

Uterine: tonic to the uterus

Vasodilator: an agent which dilates the blood vessels

Vasoconstrictor: an agent which causes narrowing of the blood vessels

Vulnerary: helps heal wounds and sores

☞ TASK

Complete the following tables by identifying the following information:

- the common name of the essential oil
- the origin of the oil (ie the part of the plant from which it is produced)
- the method of production
- list five known properties attributed to this oil

TABLE 3 *The Essential Oils*

Botanical name	Common name of essential oil	Origin	Method of production	Properties
Citrus bergamia				
Rose dameascena				
Rosemarinus officinalis				
Santalum album				

TABLE 3 *Continued*

Botanical name	Common name of essential oil	Origin	Method of production	Properties
Cananga odorata				
Piper nigrum				
Anthemis nobilis				
Salvia sclarea				

TABLE 3 *Continued*

Botanical name	Common name of essential oil	Origin	Method of production	Properties
Eucalyptus globulus				
Botswellia carteri				
Pelargonium graveolens				
Juniperus communis				

TABLE 3 *Continued*

Botanical name	Common name of essential oil	Origin	Method of production	Properties
Lavendula officinalis				
Citrus limonum				
Origanum majorana				
Mentha piperita				

? SELF-ASSESSMENT QUESTIONS

1. Why is it often said that essential oils contain the life force of the plant?

....

....

2. Why is it important to be able to recognise the botanical name of a plant in connection with an essential oil?

....

....

3. Define the following terms used to describe the therapeutic properties of essential oils:
   i)   analgesic

....

....

   ii) antispasmodic

....

....

   iii) rubefacient

....

....

   iv) febrifuge

....

....

   v)   cytophylactic

....

....

   vi) carminative

....

....

Chapter 5

BASIC CHEMISTRY FOR AROMATHERAPY

A typical essential oil is comprised from over 100 chemical compounds, and therefore has an extremely complex chemical structure. Many of the chemical compounds contained within essential oils are hard to detect and some are only present in minute quantities, making chemistry of essential oils a difficult subject to study.

The chemical make-up of an essential oil generally reflects its therapeutic effects and toxicology; in this chapter we will consider the basics of chemistry which are relevant to an aromatherapist.

- A competent aromatherapist needs a basic knowledge of chemistry, in order to understand the therapeutic properties of essential oils, along with their potential hazards.

By the end of this chapter you will be able to relate the following knowledge to your work as an aromatherapist:

- the basic principles of organic chemistry
- the classifications of essential oil compounds
- examples of common chemical constituents of essential oils
- basic chemical structures in relation to essential oils
- common analytical techniques used in the identification of the chemical constituents of an essential oil.

Before looking at the individual compounds which make up an essential oil, it is important to consider the *biosynthesis* of the plant, from which the essential oil is derived.

BASIC PRINCIPLES OF ORGANIC CHEMISTRY

Aromatherapists are the 'end users' of the essential oils, but it is important to appreciate that before they undertake their work, the plant has been produced from very simple building blocks such as light, carbon dioxide and water.

Plants have an amazing ability to synthesise chemical substances, and as mentioned above, essential oil extracted from plant materials can contain several hundred chemical constituents. It is therefore appropriate to consider the basic chemistry of carbon (C), as carbon dioxide (CO_2) is the base material used to construct all the body of plants. Carbon is a very useful element, and without it the world would be a very different place; it is at the heart of all that we are and all of the materials around us.

Essential oils are *organic* compounds, which means that they all contain the element carbon. Hydrogen, carbon and oxygen are the building blocks of essential oils, and each of these elements are themselves made up of atoms and molecules – the building blocks of the universe:

- atoms are the smallest units of any element
- molecules are the smallest units of a compound.

Compounds are formed when atoms are bonded, that is they are joined together. There are therefore two different classifications of essential oil compounds.

- **Hydrocarbons**   the first major category of compounds; these contain molecules of hydrogen and carbon only and are classified as *Terpenes.*
- **Oxygenated compounds**   the second major category of compounds; these contain hydrogen, carbon and also oxygen, and are classified under different chemical types such as *Acids, Alcohols, Aldehydes, Esters, Ketones, Lactones, Oxides* and *Phenols.*

Note: the compounds listed above are found throughout nature and are not exclusive to the world of aromatherapy and essential oils.

CHEMICAL STRUCTURE OF ESSENTIAL OILS

There are two main building blocks for the chemical structure of essential oils.

- **Isoprene unit** these structures are made up of five carbon compounds in a branched chain; see Figure 33.

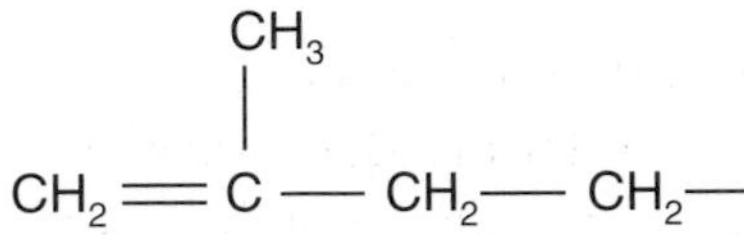

$$CH_2 = C \overset{\displaystyle CH_3}{\underset{\displaystyle |}{|}} - CH_2 - CH_2 -$$

Figure 33
Isoprene unit

- **Aromatic rings** another feature of carbon chemistry is the ability to form rings. Carbon atoms do not always join together in a branched chain, sometimes they join together in a ring, forming what is known as an aromatic ring. As the chain length increases, the potential to form rings increases. Rings can form from three carbon atoms but most are comprised of five or six atoms.

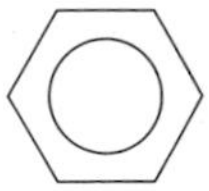

Figure 34
Aromatic ring

Organic chemistry (the chemistry of compounds containing carbon) also utilises oxygen (O), nitrogen (N), sulphur (S) as basic molecular building blocks. It is not surprising that from these basic elements it is possible to build a vast array of compounds.

TERPENES

These contain less than the maximum number of hydrogen atoms, and are referred to as 'unsaturated'. They are based on the isoprene unit, which are five-carbon compounds.

There are two main types of terpenes of interest to an aromatherapist:

- **Monoterpenes** all molecules of monoterpenes contain ten carbon units, as they are made up of two isoprene units. Common examples of monoterpenes include *limonene* (found in lemon, bergamot, neroli and orange), and *pinene* (found in cypress and eucalyptus).

  Monoterpenes are found in practically all essential oils. They have weak, uninteresting odours, are very volatile and readily oxidise.

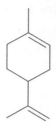

Figure 35
Limonene (monoterpene)

- **Sesquiterpenes** atoms of sesquiterpenes contain 15 carbon atoms and are therefore are made up of three isoprene units. The prefix 'sesqui' means 'one and a half'. Sesquiterpenes are a less common chemical component of essential oils. They have a strong odour and can have an important influence on the fragrance of an essential oil. Common examples of sesquiterpenes include *chamazulene* (found in the chamomiles), *bisabolene* (found in black pepper and lemon), and *caryophyllene* (found in lavender, marjoram and clary sage).

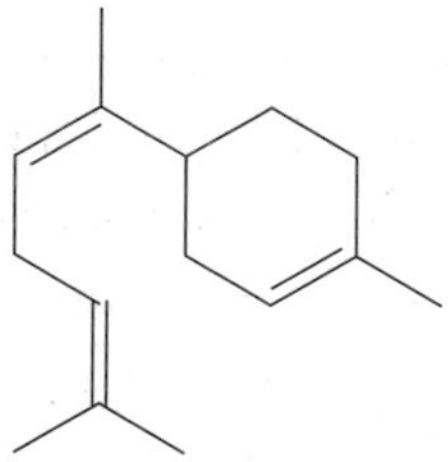

Figure 36
Bisabolene (sesquiterpene)

OXYGENATED COMPOUNDS

———————— K E Y   N O T E ————————

It is important to remember that it is the odour of oxygenated compounds and sesquiterpenes that determine the fragrance characteristics of essential oils.

ACIDS

This category of organic compounds is a rare component of essential oils. Structurally they are based on the carboxyl group and have the chemical grouping COOH.

Acids have a low volatility rate. Common examples of acids found in essential oils include *benzoic* acid in benzoin, and *geranic* acid in geranium.

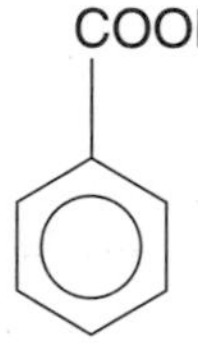

COOH

Figure 37
Benzoic acid

ALCOHOLS

These are based on monoterpenes and therefore contain ten carbon atoms. They contain the chemical functional group OH. They are referred to as terpene derivatives and are classified on the basis of which type of terpene was involved in their production:

- **Monoterpenic alcohols**   these are the most common type of alcohols found in essential oils. Examples include *linalool*, found in rosewood, and *geraniol*, found in geranium.

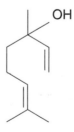

OH

Figure 38
Linalool (monoterpenic alcohol)

- **Sesquiterpenic alcohols**   these are not so common and are based on the sesquiterpenes as the name suggests. A common example of a sesquiterpenic alcohol is santalol, found in sandalwood.

ALDEHYDES

This category of organic compounds is a common essential oil component, and is based on the carbonyl group (C=O). Aldehydes have a slightly fruity odour when the odour is smelt on its own. Some aldehydes are used as skin irritants and sensitisers. Common examples of aldehydes in essential oils include: *citronellal* (found in citronella), and *citral* (found in lemongrass).

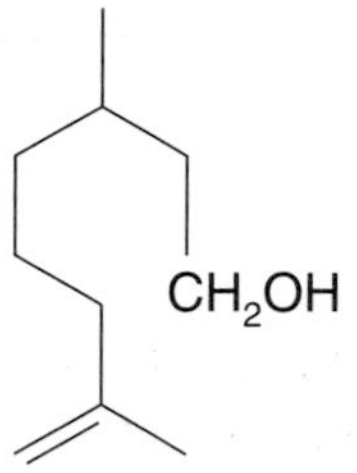

Figure 39
Citronellol (aldehyde)

ESTERS

These are very important constituents of essential oils. They are produced from the corresponding terpene alcohol and an organic acid, and are based on the carboxyl group (COOH).

The highest levels of esters are produced on the full bloom of the flower or the maturity of the fruit or plant. For example, bergamot: as the fruit begins to ripen, linalool is converted to linalyl acetate.

Common examples of esters found in essential oils include *linalyl acetate* (found in bergamot, clary sage and lavender), and *geranyl acetate* (found in sweet marjoram).

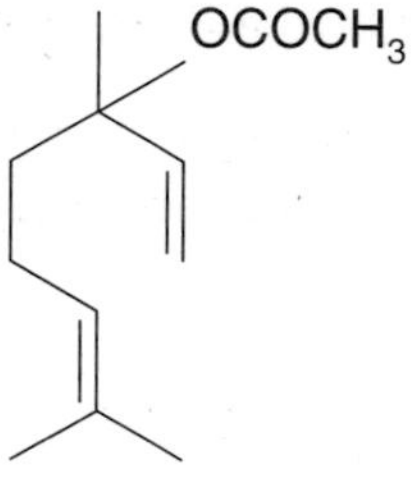

Figure 40
Linalyl acetate (ester)

KETONES

These are potentially toxic compounds and are similar in structure to aldehydes, being based on the carbonyl group (C=O).

Common examples of ketones found in essential oils include *fenchone* (found in fennel), and *camphor* (found in rosemary).

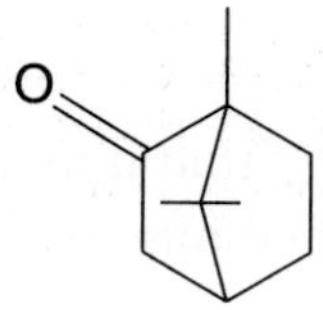

Figure 41
Camphor (ketone)

LACTONES

These are found mainly in expressed oils. A sub-group of lactones called furocoumarins are known as photo-sensitisers, and *beragptene* is the most common molecular example.

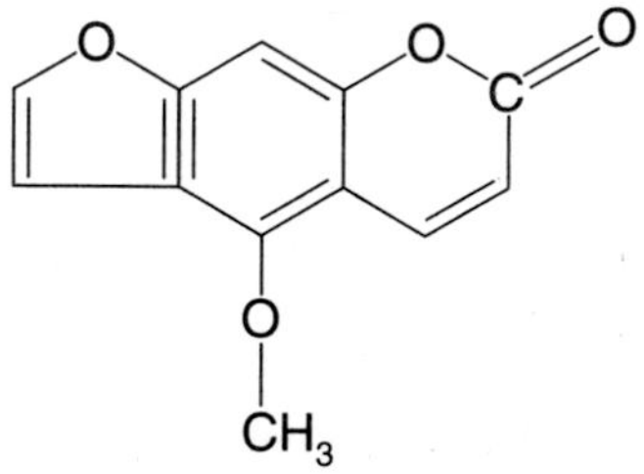

Figure 42
Bergaptene (furocoumarin-lactone)

OXIDES

These chemical compounds are rarely found in essential oils. They tend to be non-hazardous, and their chemical structure is such that the oxygen atom in the molecule is situated between two carbon atoms: C—O—C.

A common example of an oxide found in essential oils is *cineole*; in its most common form it is known as 1,8 cineole (found in eucalyptus).

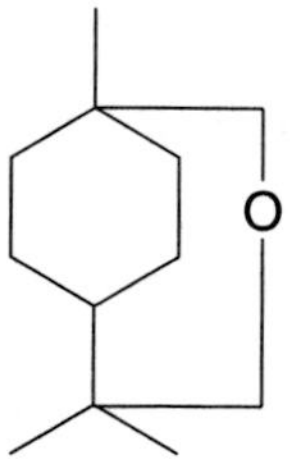

Figure 43
1,8 cineole (oxide)

PHENOLS

This category of aromatic molecules is similar to the alcohols in that they have an —OH group. In phenols, however, the OH group attaches itself to carbon in an aromatic ring.

The significance of the OH group is that it makes the phenol molecule very reactive, which explains why essential oils containing a high proportion of phenols can be irritating to the skin.

Common examples of essential oils containing phenols include: *thymol* (found in thyme), *cavacrol* (found in thyme), and *eugenol* (found in clove, cinnamon leaf, and black pepper).

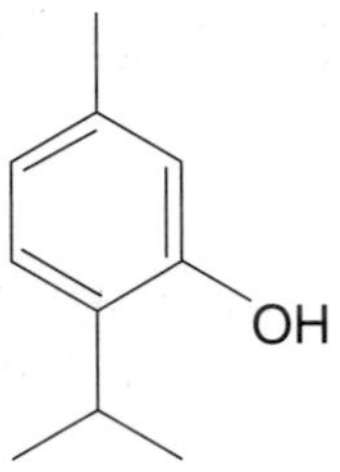

Figure 44
Thymol

SUMMARY

The two most important points are that carbon is at the heart of all essential oils, and that essential oils are made by living plants. A vast array of different compounds can be made by adding carbon atoms together, and this is increased further when we add other atoms like oxygen. The size of a molecule, its shape and the concentration of chemical constituents within the oil will therefore confer its individual and collective properties.

CHEMOTYPES

The same plant grown in different regions and under different conditions can produce essential oils of widely diverse characteristics. Variations in the chemical constituents of the oil occur and are known as *chemotypes*. The word 'chemotype' is also used to indicate oils of different chemical composition, even though they are obtained from plants which are botanically identical. Chemotypes are quite common, and essential oils will naturally vary from season to season due to the following factors:

- condition and type of soil in which the plant is grown
- region or country from which the oil was sourced
- method of extraction
- climate and conditions such as altitude.

─────────── **K E Y   N O T E** ───────────

Minor constituents or trace constituents tend to contribute more to the therapeutic qualities of the oil than do the major chemical constituents.

All chemical compounds have widely varying properties, and so it is virtually impossible to generalise about the therapeutic properties of an essential oil based only on the properties of the known chemical constituents, as you lose sight of the effects of the whole oil.

TECHNIQUES USED IN ESSENTIAL OIL ANALYSIS

It is generally accepted that the quality and 'wholeness' of an essential oil used in aromatherapy is fundamental to its therapeutic efficacy. This may be due to a number of factors:

- minor trace constituents may have therapeutic benefits
- the total benefit conferred by the whole oil is greater than the sum of its individual components
- little is known about the pharmacological actions of *all* the constituents present within an essential oil
- it is difficult to produce synthetic, simpler mixture of oils until all the individual and additive effects can be scientifically documented.

Unfortunately, there is no perfect single, analytical technique capable of identifying all the constituents chemically. However, if a reputable analytical laboratory is employed using validated methods, it is possible to 'fingerprint' an oil and compare it to a known reference.

GAS LIQUID CHROMATOGRAPHY

The technique commonly used in essential oils analysis is *Gas Liquid Chromatography* (GLC), known simply as GC. The term chromatography simply means the separation of the components of a mixture.

A Russian botanist called Michael Tswett (1872–1919) was the grandfather of modern chromatography. He discovered basic principles of column chromatography when separating plant pigments. The various pigments were separated into coloured bands, hence the name chromatography ('chromo' is Greek for colour).

Apparatus

In its most basic form, the GC apparatus comprises the following components:

- the column (typically 1–60 metres long), which is coated with a thin film of liquid
- an oven which houses the column and is capable of working within the temperature range 40–450 °C
- an injection port (the means of placing the essential oil into the column)
- a detector (the means of 'seeing' the products of the GC separation)
- a syringe (capable of injecting very small quantities, typically 0.2–5 µl)

Method

- A small amount of essential oil is injected into the port to be analysed. The amount of time taken for each chemical compound to emerge at the other end of the column (known as the retention time) is different, due to the fact that all chemical components are of different molecular size.
- The interaction of the sample components with the gas phase and the liquid phase achieves the separation.
- The quantity of each chemical component is then analysed by the detector and a peak is shown on the trace, which relates proportionally to its quantity.

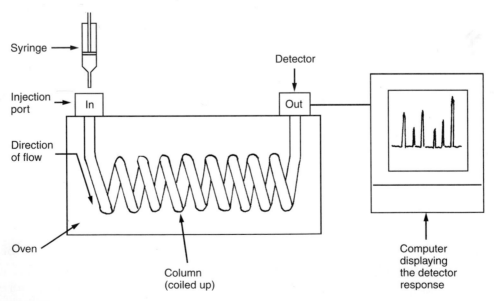

Figure 45
Gas Chromatograph

The retention time of a given component is a character of that component, and can be used to assign its identity, provided that a pure single component sample is also analysed. However, if the individual identity is not known, the analysis can be carried out and the whole chromatogram can be compared to a reference oil known to be of high quality. This process forms the basis of fingerprinting an essential oil.

The choice of detector used will influence the quality of the data collected, as some detectors can produce accurate quantitative data and others can identify the individual chemicals. Examples of two types of detector commonly used are:

- flame ionisation detector (FID)
- mass spectrometer.

Because essential oils contain several chemical functional groups and have high carbon numbers, they produce complex chromatograms.

— KEY NOTE —

Gas Chromatography is not a guaranteed test of purity, but is a comparative test; each batch tested is compared to a known reference which is the 'standard'. However, it is possible to highlight adulterants which are not evident on the 'standard'.

⚬⟶ TASK

Complete the following table to identify the following chemical compounds of essential oils.

TABLE 4: *Chemical compounds of essential oils*

Chemical compounds	Description
	Based on the carboxyl group (COOH). Rare component of essential oil; have a low volatility rate.
	Contain ten carbon atoms and the chemical functional group OH. Are referred to as terpene derivatives.
	Based on the carboxyl group ($C=O$). Commonly found as essential oil components. Some may be skin irritants and sensitisers.
	Produced from the corresponding terpene alcohol and organic acid. Based on carboxyl group (COOH). Very important constituents of essential oils.
	Based on carboxyl group (C—O), potentially toxic compounds. Similar in structure to aldehydes.
	Mainly found in expressed oil. Contains the sub group furocoumarins which are photo sensitisers.
	The structure of these compounds is that the oxygen atom in the molecule is situated between two carbon atoms C—O—C. Found rarely in essential oils.
	Contain the functional group OH which attaches itself to a carbon in an aromatic ring. Can be irritating to the skin.
	Contain ten carbon units and are therefore made up of two isoprene units. Found in practically all essential oils.
	These compounds contain 15 carbon atoms and are made up of three isoprene units. Less common component of essential oils; have an important influence on the fragrance of an essential oil.

? SELF-ASSESSMENT QUESTIONS

1. Name the chemical elements which represent the basic building blocks for essential oils.

   ....

2. State the two classifications of essential oil components, and their sub classifications.

   ....

   ....

   ....

3. Describe the two main chemical structures that form the main building blocks for essential oils.

   ....

   ....

   ....

   ....

4. What is meant by the term chemotype?

   ....

   ....

   ....

   ....

5. What is Gas Chromatography?

   ....

   ....

   ....

   ....

   ....

   ....

6. Why is it impossible to analyse all chemical constituents of an essential oil?

....

....

....

Chapter 6

~

THE PHYSIOLOGY OF AROMATHERAPY

In aromatherapy there are two ways in which essential oils may be absorbed into the bloodstream to have therapeutic effects: through the *skin,* and via the *respiratory* system. The effects of aromatherapy upon the body are so diverse because essential oils have three distinct modes of action:

- they initiate chemical changes in the body when the essential oil enters the bloodstream and reacts with hormones and enzymes
- they have a physiological effect on the systems of the body
- they have a psychological effect when the odour of the oil is inhaled.

- A competent aromatherapist needs to understand the effects of aromatherapy to appreciate the principles upon which it works.

By the end of this chapter you will be able to relate the following knowledge to your work as an aromatherapist:

- how essential oils enter the bloodstream
- the process of olfaction
- the effects of aromatherapy on the major systems of the body.

THE ABSORPTION OF ESSENTIAL OILS INTO THE BLOODSTREAM

THE SKIN

As the skin is the largest surface area for the application of essential oils, it represents the most common route for absorbing essential oils into the bloodstream for therapeutic effect.

The skin is divided into two main layers:

- the upper most superficial layer, the **epidermis** which is divided into five layers: horny layer, clear layer, granular layer, prickle cell layer and the basal cell layer
- the deeper layer, **dermis** which contains appendages such as the hair, hair follicle, sweat glands, sebaceous glands and an abundance of blood vessels which provide vital nourishment to the epidermis.

Essential oils are made up of tiny organic molecules which enable them to penetrate the skin and cross the horny layer of the epidermis, by entering the ducts of the sweat glands and hair follicles to reach the upper dermis and the capillary circulation. Essential oils are absorbed through the skin by simple

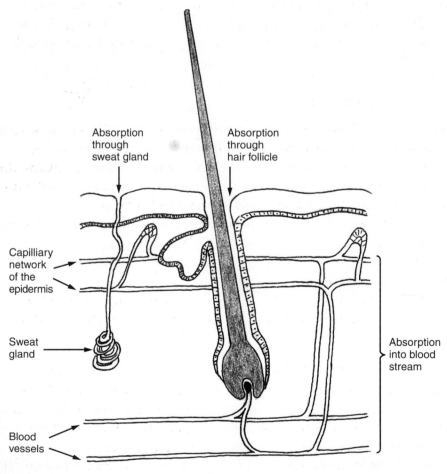

Figure 46
The absorption of essential oils into the skin

diffusion, as the skin is semi-permeable and essential oils contain constituents which are fat-soluble. The fat-soluble aromatic particles of the essential oil dissolve in the oily sebum produced by the sebaceous glands, and pass into the deeper layer of the skin (the dermis) where it is then carried by the blood and lymph vessels into the main bloodstream.

KEY NOTE

Essential oils diffuse through the skin at different rates and in certain cases can take up to 90 minutes to absorb into the bloodstream. Much depends on the surface area to which essential oils are applied, the viscosity (thickness) of the carrier oil used and the volatility rate of the essential oils.

The rate of absorption of essential oils into the skin increases greatly if the skin is damaged. Care must therefore be taken to avoid application of essential oils to broken skin, in order to prevent skin irritation and sensitisation.

Aromatherapy can help the skin in the following ways:

- Aromatherapy massage increases the absorption rate of essential oils into the skin, which penetrate the skin due to their small molecular size.
- Essential oils can help to enhance the protective function of the skin due to the fact that many essential oils are antiseptic, antibacterial and anti-fungal; for example lavender, lemon, bergamot and teatree.
- Essential oils can help the skin's cells to regenerate; examples of this are cytophylactic oils such as lavender and neroli.
- Essential oils can help to calm and soothe the skin; for example chamomile, which is anti-inflammatory.
- Essential oils can help to regulate the skin by balancing the secretion of sebum; for example geranium can be used to help both dry and oily skins.

THE RESPIRATORY SYSTEM

Respiration is one of the most basic functions of the body. Through the process of gas exchange in the lungs, essential oil particles can diffuse into the bloodstream. After passing through the nose where it has been warmed, moistened and filtered, the inhaled air (carrying aromatic particles of an essential oil) continues its journey towards the lungs. It passes through the pharynx, the larynx, the trachea and into the bronchi. Within the lungs, each bronchi divide and subdivide into smaller tubes called bronchioles. Each bronchiole then divides into alveoli – these are composed of a very thin membrane of simple epithelium, only a single layer thick so that the process of diffusion can take place.

The function of this very large expanse of film is to allow the exchange of gases between the air in the lungs and the blood in the bloodstream. Each cluster of alveoli is surrounded by a very rich network of capillaries and a moist membrane. The inhaled air carrying the essential oil particles are able to pass through these thin layers after being dissolved in the surface moisture. The capillaries surrounding the alveoli join up to form venules and arterioles, which in turn join up to form larger veins and arteries.

Therefore, any substance inhaled with the air will be involved in this complex process of gas exchange. Differing amounts of aromatic particles of essential oil will therefore be dissolved into the bloodstream from the lungs.

— KEY NOTE —

The actual amount of essential oil dissolved into the bloodstream depends on the volatility and chemical structure of the oil concerned. The absorption of essential oils into the bloodstream via the respiratory system is slower and more diffusive than any other form of application, and essential oils will not build up high levels of concentration (as long as sensible proportions are used), due to the fact that the oils are constantly being removed from the bloodstream by one or more exit pathways.

The amount of essential oil absorbed into the bloodstream can be measured by analysis of exhaled breath, blood and urine samples.

Aromatherapy massage can help the respiratory systems if suitable oils are combined which can help promote good breathing by clearing the lungs and allowing the interchange of gases to occur more efficiently.

In some cases, however, it may be more effective to use an inhalation where the physical condition would contra-indicate massage, as in the case of a client with a heavy cold. Essential oils which have an affinity for the respiratory system include:

- antiseptic oils such as lavender, bergamot, lemon, sandalwood, juniper, eucalyptus and teatree which help to prevent infections of the respiratory tract

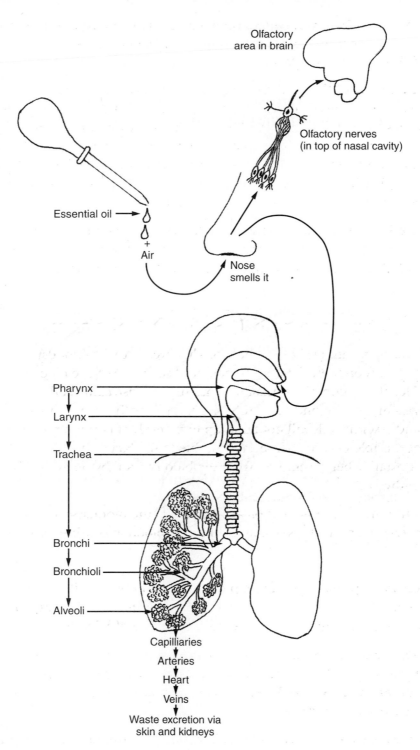

Olfactory
area in brain

Olfactory nerves
(in top of nasal cavity)

Essential oil →

+
Air

Nose
smells it

Pharynx

Larynx

Trachea

Bronchi

Bronchioli

Alveoli

Capilliaries

Arteries

Heart

Veins

Waste excretion via
skin and kidneys

Figure 47
The journey of an essential oil

- antiviral oils such as lavender, teatree and eucalyptus, which are effective in helping viral infections of the respiratory tract
- antispasmodic oils such as clary sage, peppermint and frankincense can help to calm spasms in the bronchial tubes
- expectorants which are most effective in the removal of excess phlegm include eucalyptus, peppermint and sandalwood.

THE PROCESS OF OLFACTION

- When an essential oil evaporates, the nose warms the air and the odiferous particles of the essential oil dissolve in the mucous, which covers the inner nasal cavity.
- The captivated aromatic molecules are then carried to the upper part of the nasal cavity; the site of the olfactory receptor cells, which are sensory neurones especially adapted for sensing smell.
- Delicate hair-like projections or cilia protrude from the olfactory receptor cells and are an extension of the nerve fibres connecting with the olfactory cells. These cilia have their tip in the layer of mucous and are able to detect the tiny chemical particles which enter the nose. They can pass on to the olfactory cells whatever information they have picked up about the gases passing through the nose.
- Each olfactory cell has a long nerve fibre called an axon, which leads out of the main body of the cell. When the aromatic molecules lock onto the cilia, an electrochemical message is sent to the olfactory bulb and along the olfactory tract to the limbic area of the brain, where the smell is perceived.

KEY NOTE

In most nerves of the body, the passing on of messages or impulses about the environment is done through the spinal cord and from there onto the brain. However, in the case of the olfactory cells, the nerve fibres pass through a bony plate at the top of the nose and connect directly with the area of the brain known as the olfactory bulb, which is situated in the cerebral cortex.

As the cilia are in direct contact with the source of smell and as the olfactory receptor cells connect directly with the brain, the sense of smell has a powerful and immediate effect on the body.

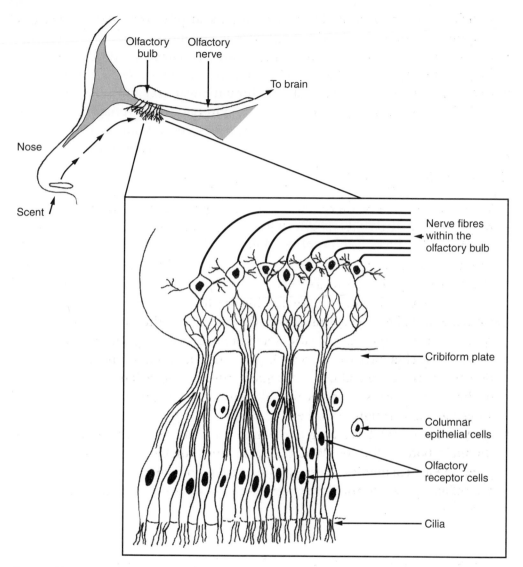

Figure 48
The theory of olfaction

THE LIMBIC SYSTEM

The limbic system is a v-shaped structure sitting on top of the brain stem, and includes the amalygda, hippocampus, part of the thalamus and the hypothalamus.

The *hippocampus* is involved in memory function and is a paired organ, with one located in each temporal lobe of the brain. In relation to olfaction, the hippocampus helps us to link that odour to its 'memory bank', to determine whether it is a familiar fragrance and if so, which related memories are brought forward into our conscious awareness. The *amygdala* are located symmetrically in the limbic system just above the hypothalamus in the anterior tip of the temporal lobes. It is thought that the amygdala works with the *hypothalamus* to mediate emotional responses; certain odours may precipitate varied emotions from pleasure to rage and aggression.

The anterior part of the limbic system is in the olfactory cortex, which explains the intimate relationship between smells and emotions.

Another part of the limbic system called the *septum pellicidum* is said to be the pleasure centre. Electrical impulses applied to this part of the brain have

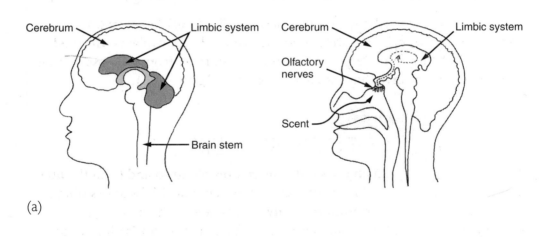

(a)

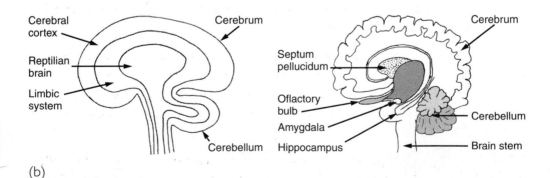

(b)

Figure 49
The limbic system

evoked happiness in depressed persons, pain relief in cancer sufferers and intensification of sexual arousal in some people.

The limbic system receives sensory input from the olfactory, visual, auditory, balance and equilibrium systems. It processes much of this input, and channels it to the cerebral cortex. It forms connections with the brain stem below and the cerebrum above and allows for a balance and integration of emotion and reason; see Figure 49(a).

The limbic system has multiple connections with the thalamus, hypothalamus and pituitary gland, which is why olfactory sensory receptors can influence endocrine function.

Functionally, the limbic system is a complex structure which has approximately 34 structures and 53 pathways. It is the major seat of our emotions, and is linked to the perception of odour, sensations of pleasure and pain, emotions like rage, fear, sadness and sexual feelings.

The complexity of the limbic systems and the direct link between the olfactory receptor cells and the limbic area of the brain explains why smell can effect an emotional response and recall a memory from the past, as scent memory is longer-term than visual memory; see Figure 49(b).

THE CIRCULATORY SYSTEM

The heart is a pump which constantly distributes blood to and from the lungs and all around the body in a double circuit. All chemical substances which need to be transported around the body are carried by the blood, eg hormones. The blood circulates around the body at a surprisingly fast speed, taking about a half minute to complete a circuit. This means that when substances such as essential oil particles are dissolved into the bloodstream, they can take effect very quickly.

Some essential oils have affinities with certain organs or systems, and will have a special effect on that organ or system when at that point in its circulating journey. The oils will be either wholly or partly deposited in any organs for which they have a special affinity; others will exercise a more general effect.

Whatever part of the essential oil is left after its therapeutic work in the body has been done, will be excreted by one path or another. It may be passed out of the body in urine or faeces, excreted through the skin as sweat or returned to the lungs to be exhaled with the breath.

How aromatherapy can help the circulatory system

Combining essential oils with aromatherapy massage techniques can help our circulatory system to work more efficiently by stimulating the circulation, but can also help to relieve tension (which puts undue stress on the system and restricts the blood flow). For example:

- lavender is a heart sedative and can help to reduce palpitations and lower blood pressure
- lemon is a tonic to the circulation and can help to liquefy the blood
- neroli can aid a poor circulation due to its depurative effect (blood cleaning).

THE LYMPHATIC SYSTEM

The lymphatic system has three main functions:

- **Drainage of excess fluid from the body cells and tissues**   extra cellular fluid from the tissue is absorbed into the lymphatic vessels and is carried away to the lymph nodes to be cleansed before entering the bloodstream via the subclavian veins.
- **Fighting infection**   the lymph nodes manufacture lymphocytes and generate antibodies which help to ingest and neutralise invading bacteria. The lymph nodes act as filtering stations and are densely packed with the lymphocytes, which ingest foreign bodies as the lymph (colourless fluid containing white blood cells) passes through the nodes.
- **Absorption and distribution of fat soluble nutrients**   upon reaching the small intestine, the products of fat digestion pass into the lymphatic system via intestinal lymphatic called the lacteals.

Aromatherapy places particular importance upon the lymphatic system in that it helps to facilitate several actions:

- stimulate immunity
- encourage the flow of lymph from the tissues and into the circulatory system
- prevent oedema
- reduce the viscosity of blood
- reduce generalised swelling in the tissues
- stimulate the absorption of waste material from the tissues.

Aromatherapy can help the lymphatic system in the following ways:

- diuretic essential oils help to accelerate lymph and tissue fluid circulation, eg fennel, lemon, juniper and geranium
- essential oils help stimulate the circulatory system, eg black pepper, rosemary and ginger
- essential oils can help to increase the production of white blood cells to stimulate immunity, eg bergamot, lavender, lemon, chamomile, rosemary and thyme
- all essential oils are antiseptic and bactericidal to some extent, but chamomile, lavender, lemon, clove, sandalwood and teatree are probably the most effective in relation to these properties.

THE ENDOCRINE SYSTEM

The endocrine system is a highly sophisticated system of communication and co-ordination, which governs many body processes.

The endocrine glands which make up the system each secrete chemicals (hormones) into the bloodstream. These chemicals can influence parts of the body which are often quite distant from the point of secretion. The main endocrine glands include the following:

- Pituitary gland
- Thyroid gland
- Parathyroid glands
- Adrenal glands
- The islets of langerhans
- Ovaries
- Testes.

There are many similarities between an essential oil and a hormone:

- both contain chemical compounds
- both are transported by the bloodstream
- both can help to regulate body processes
- both affect our physical and psychological well-being
- both can have a direct or an indirect effect on the body.

Essential oils appear to act on the endocrine system and on various body functions regulated by the endocrine system, in two ways:

- directly
- indirectly.

DIRECT EFFECT

Certain essential oils contain plant hormones or *phytohormones*. They can act on the body in the same way as a hormone, in that they directly affect a target organ or tissue. For example, the essential oil of fennel contains a form of oestrogen in its structure and therefore can be effective for female problems such as pre-menstrual syndrome and the menopause; rose and jasmine have a direct effect on the reproductive system and have been used to help stimulate contraction of the uterus in labour, as well as helping with female reproductive problems.

INDIRECT EFFECT

Essential oils can influence the hormone secretion of the various glands. They act as triggers, stimulating the production of a hormone or a balancing agent which may either help to raise or reduce the amount of a hormone that is being produced, thereby restoring the endocrine system to a more balanced state. For example, geranium helps to stimulate the adrenal cortex, which will indirectly influence the secretion of the corticoid hormones; clary sage, lavender and ylang ylang all help to lower blood pressure.

THE NERVOUS SYSTEM

The nervous system is the main communication system for the body and works intimately with the endocrine system to regulate body processes. It has two main divisions:

- the *central nervous system*, which is the control centre and consists of a two-way communication system of the brain and the spinal cord
- the *peripheral* system, consisting of nerves which carry messages to and from the central nervous system.

THE CENTRAL NERVOUS SYSTEM

The functional unit of the nervous system is a neurone or nerve, and there are two main types of nerve impulses:

- sensory nerves which receive stimuli from sensory organs and receptors, and transmit the impulses to the spinal cord and brain
- motor nerves which conduct nerve impulses away from the central nervous system towards muscles and glands, to stimulate them into action.

─────────── **KEY NOTE** ───────────

In aromatherapy massage, the sensory stimulus of touch and pressure will be received by the sensory receptors in the skin, and smell will be received by the olfactory receptors cells in the top of the nasal cavity.

Sensory impulses are important for the success of aromatherapy treatment as they will convey both the aroma and the touch associated with massage, along the nerve pathways up the central nervous system to the brain, where they will be perceived by the limbic system.

The most important areas of the brain for aromatherapy are therefore:
- **the olfactory bulb**   in the cerebral cortex, perceives the aroma
- **the limbic system**   known as the 'smell brain', related to emotions and memory
- **the hypothalamus**   regulates other body functions through its control of the endocrine system and autonomic nervous system.

─────────── **KEY NOTE** ───────────

The hypothalamus is a structure at the base of the brain and is linked with the rest of the brain and the pituitary gland by a complex network of nerve pathways. It serves as an interface between the mind, the nervous system and endocrine systems.

It controls hunger, thirst, temperature, sexual response and is also closely involved with our emotions and sleep patterns.

THE PERIPHERAL NERVOUS SYSTEM

The peripheral nervous system is made up of the parts of the nervous system outside of the brain and spinal cord. It comprises of:

- 31 pairs of spinal nerves
- 12 pairs of cranial nerves
- the autonomic nervous system.

The 31 pairs of spinal nerves pass out of the spinal cord. Each has two thin branches which link it with the autonomic nervous system. Spinal nerves receive sensory impulses from the body and transmit motor signals to specific regions of the body. By stimulating the spinal nerves through aromatherapy massage, communication can be made with many of the organs of the body (respiratory, digestive, sensory, urinary and reproductive) and any blockages and weaknesses in the nerve pathways can be assisted to clear.

Aromatherapy can help the nervous system by:

- reducing nervous tension and helping stress-related conditions
- inducing relaxation
- stimulating the nerves to clear congestion in the nerves and thereby improve the functioning of related organs and tissues.

Examples of essential oils which have an affinity for the nervous system include the following:

- bergamot, chamomile, jasmine, lavender, neroli, sweet marjoram and ylang ylang are sedatives and have a calming effect on the central nervous system.
- peppermint, lemon and rosemary have a stimulating effect on the nervous system.
- chamomile, clary sage, juniper, lavender, marjoram and rosemary are nerve tonics and help to strengthen the nervous system.

THE MUSCULO-SKELETAL SYSTEM

Aromatherapy can be effective on both the muscular and skeletal system in the following ways:

- Analgesic essential oils such as lavender, chamomile, rosemary and marjoram can aid the relaxation of tense and painful muscle fibres, tendons and ligaments.
- Rufebacient essential oils such as rosemary and black pepper can assist in increasing the blood supply to the soft tissues, bones and joints, helping to promote flexibility and reduce the risk of injury.
- Anti-inflammatory essential oils such as chamomile and lavender can help to reduce inflammation around joints.
- Detoxifying essential oils such as lemon and juniper can assist in eliminating waste products such as lactic acid and uric acid from the tissues.

--- **KEY NOTE** ---

In cases where an area may be too painful to massage, it may be more preferable to use a compress to help reduce inflammation, swelling and pain.

✏ **TASK**

Complete the following table to illustrate which essential oils may be effective for the following systems.

TABLE 5: *Essential oils and systems of the body*

Type of	Essential oils which may be effective on the system
Skin	
Respiratory	
Blood Circulation	
Lymphatic	

TABLE 5: *Continued*

Type of	Essential oils which may be effective on the system
Endocrine	
Nervous	
Musculo-skeletal	

❓ SELF-ASSESSMENT QUESTIONS

1. Explain briefly the two main ways in which essential oils are absorbed into the bloodstream for therapeutic effect.

   ....

   ....

   ....

   ....

   ....

   ....

   ....

....
....
....
....
....

2. List the principal parts of the olfactory system.

....
....
....
....
....
....

3. Briefly explain the process of olfaction.

....
....
....
....
....
....
....

4. How can a smell stimulate an emotional response within the brain?

....
....
....
....
....

5. State five similarities between essential oils and hormones.

....

....

....

....

....

....

....

Chapter 7

───────◇───────

THE AROMATHERAPY CONSULTATION

A consultation is a very important part of the whole aromatherapy treatment, and should be holistic in its approach. The initial consultation allows the aromatherapist to determine as far as possible the client's needs and will establish whether treatment is appropriate or whether referral to another professional should be the next course of action.

From the information elicited from the consultation, the aromatherapist may then select and blend oils based upon the client's physical and emotional condition, and plan a treatment to suit their needs.

- A competent aromatherapist will develop good communication and client-handling skills, in order to elicit as much information as possible, while at the same time building a good rapport and level of trust with a client.

By the end of this chapter you will be able to relate the following knowledge to your work as an aromatherapist:

- relevant factors to be discussed during an aromatherapy consultation to identify clients' needs
- how to keep full and accurate records
- professional etiquette in handling referral data
- guidelines on detailing case studies.

THE PURPOSE OF A CONSULTATION

A consultation is the first line of communication between the client and the aromatherapist, and best results are gained through co-operation and good communication between both parties. The purpose of an aromatherapy consultation is to enable the aromatherapist to:

- establish whether the client is suitable for treatment or whether a medical referral is required
- establish the need for any special care, which may involve an adaptation of treatment and oils used
- develop a good rapport with the client
- explain what aromatherapy is, along with its benefits
- identify the objectives of the treatment
- agree a treatment plan with the client to suit their needs
- answer the client's questions and allay any fears regarding the nature of the treatment.

An aromatherapy treatment should always commence with a consultation. The aromatherapist will be aware of the client's characteristics and body language from the moment the client walks in; everything will contribute to the overall picture of the client.

A skilled aromatherapist will also be an accomplished listener. S/he will listen carefully to what the client says and empathise with their problems, while also helping them to accept responsibility for their problems, and to accept help from the aromatherapist.

Aromatherapists as professionals must do their utmost to ascertain the nature of any ailment or condition prior to treatment. If any doubt exists about the health of the client and their suitability to treatment, they should be referred to their medical practitioner.

KEY NOTE

If a consultation has been undertaken and a specific medical condition arises, it should be explained to the client why aromatherapy may not be carried out without a doctor's referral.

If the client gives permission, a letter may be sent to the client's GP asking for further information regarding the client's condition, and whether aromatherapy treatment may progress.

The client may wish to take the letter to their GP directly or may wish for the aromatherapist to communicate directly with the doctor by post.

A record of all communication should be made on the consultation noting the date the letter was sent and the date it was received.

NO treatment should be carried out until medical approval has been granted.

If the GP gives approval, it is professional etiquette to keep him/her informed of the progress of the client, along with any results arising from the treatment given.

The information elicited from the consultation will form the basis upon which the aromatherapist makes a selection of appropriate oils to use for treatment. It is essential, therefore, that the client is prepared to disclose any relevant information regarding their health and condition, to enable the aromatherapist to choose suitable oils and avoid those which may be contra-indicated.

Although the initial consultation is generally the most important one for establishing the main factors relating to the client, it is important to remember that consultations are ongoing. Each treatment should be planned individually on each treatment occasion, to ensure that all client details which may affect the treatment are up to date.

CONFIDENTIALITY

It is very important that records of all consultations are kept confidentially. This should be explained to clients in order to reassure them. Maintaining client confidentiality will show a high degree of professionalism and will prevent embarrassment and loss of client loyalty.

During a consultation, the aromatherapist will need to ask the client personal questions. When asking questions of a personal nature, it is important for the aromatherapist to maintain a polite, sensitive and professional manner and it should be stressed to clients that the information asked is necessary to help establish how you can help them.

When carrying out a consultation, it is important to seat yourselves in a comfortable area, preferably out of earshot of others, and to remember to maintain eye contact throughout. Try to turn the questions into more of a chat rather than sounding as if you are merely completing a form, as this will personalise the treatment and relax the client. If you ask the questions in an open way, you will generally find that clients are more co-operative with their responses.

> ——————— **KEY NOTE** ———————
>
> Whilst the aromatherapist should always have the client's best interests at heart, it is important to remain positive about the treatment and not to become personally involved with the client's problems.
>
> Aromatherapists must remain professionally detached from the client's problems at all times, otherwise they may become unable to help them.

THE CONSULTATION FORM

Consultation forms are used to record information regarding the client's health, both past and present, and will highlight the client's present condition in order to establish the basis upon which the treatment will be formed. See pages 118–20 for a sample consultation form.

The main factors to be considered during the consultation include:

MEDICAL HISTORY

It is important to know the client's medical history, as certain conditions may contra-indicate or restrict aromatherapy treatment, and a GP referral may be needed prior to the commencement of treatment.

CURRENT MEDICAL TREATMENT

If the client is under GP or hospital care, a GP referral will be necessary in order to establish the nature of the treatment and how it might affect the proposed aromatherapy treatment.

MEDICATION

It is necessary to ascertain the type of allopathic medicine prescribed. GP referral may be necessary, as certain medications are incompatible with aromatherapy and may cause unpleasant side effects.

GENERAL HEALTH

It is important that the client's general health and well-being is discussed during the consultation. This may involve their general immunity, energy levels, stress levels and sleep patterns, which will all contribute to the overall picture of the client.

EMOTIONAL STATE

As our emotions can have a profound effect on the way we feel, it is important to establish the client's emotional state prior to treatments as this may affect the selection of oils chosen. For example, they may wish to feel uplifted or calmed and relaxed.

LIFESTYLE

A client's lifestyle will play an important part in their general well-being. Information regarding the client's job and home circumstances will often reflect the type of lifestyle they lead. Exercise undertaken is included under the heading of general lifestyle; if the client undertakes no exercise, it could lead to fluid retention, a reduction in the efficiency of the lymphatic system and poor energy levels.

DIET AND NUTRITION

It is important to have information regarding a typical daily diet of the client (including fluid levels), to ensure that they are eating the correct amount of nutrients for correct body functioning. Malnutrition can put stress onto the body and lead to increased stress levels and irritability.

Alcohol consumption and smoking levels are important factors to know about, as these will also affect the health of the client.

HOBBIES AND RELAXATION

It is important to discuss whether a client has time for a hobby and relaxation. By having an interest in a hobby, a client is able to relax and unwind, which gives the mind and body a chance to escape everyday stresses and to recuperate.

RECORD KEEPING

It is very important to ensure that a full consultation is undertaken with each client and that a record of each treatment is kept. All records should be kept confidentially and be accurate and up to date.

The treatment record should include the following information:

- results from last treatment (if applicable)
- proposed treatment plan (should take account of length of treatment, areas for treatment, number of treatments and the availability of the client)
- treatment objective
- essential oils blended and reasons for use
- dilution of essential oils used
- after care given

(list continued on page 122)

AROMATHERAPY CONSULTATION FORM

Client Note

The following information is required for your safety and to benefit your health. Whilst essential oils and massage are totally safe when administered professionally by an aromatherapist, there are certain contra-indications which require special attention.

The following details will be treated in the strictest of confidence. It may, however, be necessary for you to consult your GP before any aromatherapy treatment can be given.

Date of initial consultation: Client ref. no.:

GENERAL

Name:

Address:

Telephone Number – Daytime: Evening:

Date of Birth: Occupation:

MEDICAL

Name of Doctor: Surgery:

Address: Tel No.:

Medical Details

Do you have or have you ever suffered with any of the following:

Circulatory disorder
Heart condition
High or low Blood Pressure
Thrombosis
Varicose Veins
Epilepsy
Diabetes
Dysfunction of the Nervous System
Recent haemorrhage or swelling
Recent operation / fracture / sprain
Abdominal complaint
Skin Disorder
A potentially fatal or terminal condition (ie cancer)

Female Clients

Is it possible that you may be pregnant?
If pregnant, how many months (any history of miscarriage)?
Are you currently menstruating?
Number of pregnancies (with dates)
Are you currently under GP / Hospital care?

Current medical treatment

Current medication (list dosages)

GP Referral Required?   Yes (   ) No (   )

Clearance form sent   Yes (   )   No (   )   Date:
Clearance form received   Yes (   )   No (   )   Date:

GENERAL HEALTH

Is your general immunity/health   GOOD / AVERAGE / POOR

Would you say your energy levels are   HIGH / AVERAGE / LOW

Would you consider your stress levels to be   HIGH / AVERAGE / LOW

Sleep patterns?

HEALTH RELATED PROBLEMS
Do you suffer with any of the following:

Skin Complaints ie
Allergies / Dermatitis / Eczema / Psoriasis / Other?

Problems with Circulation, Muscles, Nerves and Joints ie
Arthritis / Muscular Aches and pains / Chilblains / Oedema / Rheumatism / Sciatica / Other?

Respiratory problems ie
Asthma / Breathing difficulties / Bronchitis / Throat infection / Sinusitis / Colds / Flu / Other?

Digestive problems ie
Constipation / Indigestion / Colitis / Candida / Other?

Urinary problems ie
Cystitis / Thrush / Fluid Retention / Other?

Nervous / Stress related problems ie
Anxiety / Depression / Headaches / Migraine / Insomnia / Nervous tension / Other?

Female Clients
Pre-menstrual Tension / Menopausal problems / Problems with periods?

Is there any other problem that has not been mentioned that you would like help with as part of this treatment?

Summary of client's main presenting problem/s:

LIFESTYLE

Typical daily diet:

Number of glasses of water consumed daily:

Number of cups of tea / coffee per day:

Vitamins / minerals taken:

Typical weekly alcohol consumption   Do you smoke? If so how many daily?

Type of exercise undertaken (and how frequently)

Do you have any hobbies? Do you relax regularly, if so how?

Have you tried aromatherapy or any other complementary therapies before?
(state when and what the results were)

Are you currently having any complementary treatment? (give details)

CLIENT DECLARATION

I declare that the information I have given is correct and as far as I am aware I can undertake treatment with this establishment without any adverse effects. I have been fully informed about contra-indications and I am therefore willing to proceed with the treatment.

Client's Signature: Date:

Therapist's Signature:

Notes

Figure 50
A sample consultation form

AROMATHERAPY TREATMENT SHEET

Client's ref. number .... **Date of Treatment** ....

Feedback from last treatment (if applicable)

Current state of health / well being

TREATMENT PLAN

TREATMENT OBJECTIVE

RANGE OF AROMATHERAPY MASSAGE MOVEMENTS
lymph drainage / pressure points / neuromuscular / effleurage / petrissage / connective tissue

ESSENTIAL OILS SELECTED (stating reasons for choice AND number of drops of each)

% DILUTION BLENDED

CARRIER OIL/S USED (state mls of oil used)

EVALUATION OF AROMATHERAPY MASSAGE
Visual & Tactile Analysis

Areas of Pain

Areas of Tension

Flare Reaction

Skin Type

Circulation

Muscle Tone

HOME CARE ADVICE GIVEN

OUTCOME OF TREATMENT

SUGGESTED PLANS FOR FUTURE TREATMENT

Therapist's signature and brief evaluation

Figure 51
A sample treatment sheet

- home care advice given (including blend of oils given to the client for home use)
- outcome of treatment with regard to effectiveness
- recommendations for future treatments.

See page 121 for a sample treatment sheet.

━━━━━ K E Y N O T E ━━━━━

It is very important to review the client's treatment plan at regular intervals, along with the oils used. Care should be taken to avoid using the same blend of oils for an extended period of time, to avoid the client building up sensitivity to an oil or oils used. Due to the diversity of properties of essential oils, there will always be a suitable alternative, preventing the need to use the same oils each time.

 TASK

Practise carrying out detailed consultations on clients in preparation for an aromatherapy treatment. These may form part of your portfolio of evidence, to compile aromatherapy case studies.

Each consultation you carry out should include the following information in relation to the client:

- personal details
- medical history
- current medical treatment
- medication
- emotional state
- lifestyle and diet
- reasons for treatment.

GUIDELINES FOR CASE STUDIES

A client case study is a record of a series of treatments which have been undertaken on a client and have been evaluated for their effectiveness.

A complete case study will generally consist of the following parts:

- A general introduction to the client to include their background information such as present condition, lifestyle and emotional state, along with the main treatment objectives.

- A completed consultation form which is detailed and elicits their physical and emotional state, and all other relevant factors.
- A record of all treatments undertaken and an evaluation of their effectiveness.
- Summary and conclusion after a course of treatments have been given. You may ask the client to complete a feedback sheet or give a testimonial.

KEY NOTE

Remember that client case studies contain confidential information, therefore it is important to obtain the client's written permission that they do not object to details being kept in your portfolio.

? SELF-ASSESSMENT QUESTIONS

1. State two important reasons for undertaking a consultation prior to aromatherapy treatment.

....

....

....

2. Why is it important to keep full and accurate records on aromatherapy treatments given for each client?

....

....

....

....

3. State ten factors which should be discussed with a client during a consultation for aromatherapy.

....

....

....

....
....
....
....
....
....
....
....
....

4. Explain the procedure and etiquette for dealing with referral data for aromatherapy treatments.

....
....
....
....
....
....
....
....
....
....

Chapter 8

~

BLENDING IN AROMATHERAPY

The art of blending essential oils is one of the most creative parts of an aromatherapy practice. When essential oils are blended together, their molecules combine to form a *synergy* so that the combination of essential oils or the 'whole' becomes more than the sum of its individual parts.

The art of true aromatherapy therefore lies in selecting and blending oils to create *synergistic* blends.

- A competent aromatherapist will have a thorough knowledge of the therapeutic properties of essential oils, and will be able to select and blend oils individually for each client.

By the end of this chapter you will be able to relate the following knowledge to your work carried out as an aromatherapist:

- the principles of synergy and blending
- factors to be considered when blending essential oils
- quantities and proportions when blending essential oils
- the therapeutic properties and uses of carrier oils.

SYNERGY

When two or more oils are blended together, the chemistry of the oils combine with one another to create an entirely new substance whose properties as a whole add up to more than the sum of its individual parts. By blending together mutually enhancing oils, the interaction of the various molecular components creates a synergistic blend which is more powerful than using an individual oil on its own.

Furthermore, the principle of synergy allows the therapist to be accurate in providing treatments by taking into account all factors relating to the client, both physical and psychological and creating a blend to suit their individual needs and condition.

The principle of synergy was strongly advocated by Marguerite Maury when she introduced the idea of the 'individual prescription' in the 1950s.

KEY NOTE

The principle of synergy is context-dependent, which means that a successful synergistic blend created for one client may be wholly inappropriate for another client. A synergistic blend therefore treats the person in a *holistic* way by taking account of all aspects of that person, rather than treating them for an isolated condition.

BLENDING

Blending essential oils is an individual skill and there are many ways in which it can be undertaken.

Firstly, in order to be able to blend essential oils successfully you will need to study the therapeutic properties of the oils to understand their effects and their individual characters (see Chapter 4), as well as having personal experience of using the oils.

Personal experimentation is the only way to learn, as essential oils possess an array of therapeutic possibilities which can be blended into endless combinations.

There are many factors to consider when blending essential oils:

PROPORTIONS

When blending it is important to remember that essential oils are very powerful and concentrated substances; it is often the minute proportions of an essential oil that can effect the healing process.

For aromatherapy massage, a dilution of 2% of essential oil to carrier oil is usually recommended.

An easy way of remembering the number of essential oil drops to carrier oil is to divide the mls of carrier oil you are using, by two. For example, if you are using 30 ml of carrier oil, you could add *up to* 15 drops of essential oil to make your blend.

KEY NOTE

In aromatherapy, it does not always follow that the more you use, the better the effect will be; the reverse is often the case. Some aromatherapists may use more or less than a 2% dilution to achieve the desired effects, but the most important overriding factor is that the proportions used are sensible and are within safety guidelines to avoid undesired effects.

It is also important to consider the odour intensity of the oils being used as some may predominate so will need to be used in small amounts to create a balanced blend.

CLIENT TYPE

The type of client to be treated will always influence the essential oils blended. For children and pregnant women it is recommended that a 1% dilution is used and there are several essential oils which should not be used (see Chapter 2).

AREA BEING TREATED

Unless the client has a very sensitive skin, it is usual to use a 2% dilution of essential oils for therapeutic body work. However, when working on sensitive areas such as the face, it is recommended that a 1% dilution is used.

Do remember also to consider your choice of oils when working on the face; some may be too stimulating, for example marjoram and black pepper.

COMPATIBILITY

Certain essential oils are mutually enhancing and will blend well together, whereas some have an inhibiting effect on each other. Personal experimentation is the only way of finding which oils blend well together, but it is worth considering that botanical families of oils blend well with each other; for example, members of the herb family (lavender, marjoram, rosemary) blend well with citrus (lemon, orange, bergamot) and flowers (rose, ylang ylang, jasmine).

NOTES

The classification of essential oils into notes originates from the perfumery industry, where it is said that a well-balanced perfume contains a top, middle and base note. This principle is not used in quite the same way for aromatherapy as for perfumery, although it may be useful to take account of notes to ensure that the blend you create is well-balanced from an aesthetic point of view.

- Top notes are the fastest acting essences and give the first impression in a blend as they are highly volatile.
- Middle notes are less volatile and usually form the heart of the blend.
- Base notes are the least volatile and act as blend fixatives to make the aroma last longer.

AESTHETICS

Although we are principally blending essential oils for therapeutic reasons, it is a good idea to take into account the aesthetics of the aroma to ensure you create a balanced blend. Smell is a very powerful sense and if the aroma of the blend is not pleasing to the client, the overall objectives may not be met as the client might not be able to relax and enjoy the full benefits of the treatment.

It is therefore very important to consider the odour intensity of the oils you intend to blend, as some oils are highly odiferous and may need to be toned down with other, less powerful and more balancing oils.

CLIENT PREFERENCE

The client's choice of aroma is often very personal, as blends react with the individual chemistry of a person's skin to create an entirely unique aroma.

COST

It is important to blend only as much as you need for an individual treatment to ensure cost-effectiveness. Treatment is not always improved by adding several essential oils, and it is wasteful to use several oils for the sake of blending if fewer oils would fit the overall purpose.

By using a maximum of three or four essential oils to a blend, you will keep in touch with the individual aroma and qualities of the oils as you start to create synergistic blends.

TREATMENT OBJECTIVE AND INDIVIDUAL NEEDS OF CLIENT

As you are creating a synergistic blend it is essential to take account of the client's predominant problems (both physical and emotional) along with an overall treatment objective, to ensure the client's needs are being met. For example, does the client need general relaxation physically but an uplift emotionally?

CLIENT'S SKIN TYPE

The client's skin type may often influence your choice of essential oils. For example, if your client suffers from skin problems, the dilution and type of oils must be carefully selected to avoid adverse skin reactions.

VARIATIONS IN BLENDING

There are many accepted variations in blending techniques which will often be unique to the person creating the blend. A good analogy is to imagine following a recipe book, while at the same time adding in one's own interpretation or ingredients to make it unique.

Some aromatherapists use dowsing or crystals to assist them in their selection of oils for a client, while others use the Eastern principle of yin (being calming and relaxing) and yang (being stimulating). Certain aromatherapists are guided by their intuition, based upon their knowledge of the therapeutic effects and characteristics of each oil.

When blending, your nose is generally the best guide, combined with personal experimentation and experience.

Whichever method of blending is used, these important factors must be considered:

- Is the blend of oils created acceptable to the client?
- Does the blend meet with the treatment objective?
- Has the blend been created synergistically, taking into account all relevant factors relating to the client?
- Are the proportions used within safe limits?

KEY NOTE

Once you begin to blend, it becomes a creative experience. In the early stages it is a good idea to keep a blending notebook detailing the oils used, proportion used and whether it was pleasing and therapeutically beneficial.

PROPERTIES AND USES OF CARRIER OILS

In order to aid their absorption into the bloodstream, essential oils are carried by base or vegetable carrier oils. Carrier oils are commonly referred to as fixed oils, as they act as blending or stabilising agents for the essential oils. In addition, they have therapeutic benefits of their own which can enhance the effectiveness of the blend.

Carrier oils used in aromatherapy should preferably be unrefined or cold pressed. The refining process of vegetable oils is undesirable in the practice of aromatherapy, as the oils are produced by intense heat which has a destructive effect on the aroma, colour and its natural constituents (ie vitamins, minerals and enzymes).

Unrefined oils are superior in comparison as they retain their natural constituents, which are therapeutically beneficial for the skin and the body's systems. The main method used for extracting vegetable carrier oils is cold or warm pressing: the oil seed, nut or kernel is heated at a low temperature to help release the oil, and is then put through a cold press.

The choice of carrier oil used in a blend will be primarily dependent on the client's skin type and the therapeutic objectives of the treatment.

COMMON CARRIER OILS USED IN AROMATHERAPY

APRICOT KERNEL

KEY NOTE

Apricot kernel is generally too expensive to use on its own so it may be blended with other less expensive carriers such as grapeseed and sweet almond. It is very effective for therapeutic massage and is light enough for facial massage.

Botanical name: *Prunus armenica*
Source: extracted from the seed kernel of the fruit
Colour: pale yellow
Contains: vitamins and minerals, notably vitamin A
Therapeutic properties: very easily absorbed, nourishing and soothing
Skin types suitable for: all skin types, especially dry, sensitive, mature and inflamed

AVOCADO

> ### KEY NOTE
>
> As this oil is fairly viscous, highly odorous and relatively expensive, use as a 10% addition to another lighter carrier.

Botanical name: *Persea americana*
Source: cold pressed from the flesh of the avocado fruit
Colour: dark green
Therapeutic properties: soothing, relieves itching, highly penetrative. Contains protein, lecithin, essential fatty acids, vitamins A, B and D
Skin types suitable for: all skin types, especially dry, dehydrated and sensitive

CALENDULA (POT MARIGOLD)

> ### KEY NOTE
>
> This oil is especially gentle and soothing for use with children, babies and those with sensitive skin.

Botanical name: *Calendula officinalis*
Source: macerated from the flowers
Colour: orange-yellow
Therapeutic properties: anti-inflammatory, astringent, softening and soothing on the skin, healing
Skin types suitable for: all skin types, especially dry and sensitive

EVENING PRIMROSE

> ### KEY NOTE
>
> This oil is reputed to be effective for menopausal problems and pre-menstrual syndrome. It is a very expensive oil so use as 10% dilution to other carrier oils; alternatively, buy in capsule form and add one or two capsules to the blend.

Botanical name: *Oenothera biennis*
Source: extracted from the seeds
Colour: pale yellow
Therapeutic properties: soothing and nourishing, reputed to help accelerate

healing in the body. Contains polyunsaturated fatty acids and is rich in linoleic acid
Skin types suitable for: all skin types, especially dry

GRAPESEED

KEY NOTE

This oil has a very light texture and is effective for general massage purposes. It can therefore be used on its own as a carrier, but is more commonly used as the main basic oil and other oils with more nutrients are added to it.

Botanical name: *Vitis vinifera*
Source: heat extracted from the grape pips of the fruit
Colour: pale green
Therapeutic properties: gentle emollient. Contains linoleic acid, protein and a small proportion of vitamin E. Free from cholesterol
Skin types suitable for: all skin types

HAZELNUT

KEY NOTE

This oil is quickly absorbed for massage purposes and can be used as 100% carrier, although it does tend to be expensive.

Botanical name: *Corylus avellana*
Source: extracted from hazelnuts
Colour: yellow
Therapeutic properties: has a slightly astringent effect on the skin and is stimulating to the circulation. Good penetrative qualities. Contains oleic acid (monosaturated fatty acid) and linoleic acid (polyunsaturated fatty acid). Contains vitamin E
Skin types suitable for: all skin types, especially oily or combination skins

JOJOBA

KEY NOTE

This oil is light and fine in texture and is very effective for facial and body massage. As it is rich and expensive, it may be added to other carriers or used on its own.

Botanical name: *Simmondsia chinensis*
Source: extracted from the bean of the plant
Colour: yellow (liquid wax)
Therapeutic properties: anti-inflammatory, highly penetrative. Its chemical structure resembles sebum and contains a waxy substance which mimics collagen. Rich in vitamin E, protein and minerals. Natural moisturiser
Skin types suitable for: all skin types including oily, combination, acne skins and inflamed skins

MACADAMIA NUT

KEY NOTE

This oil has become a very popular carrier in aromatherapy due to its nutritive properties.

Botanical name: *Macadamia integrifolia* and *Macadamia ternifolia*
Source: warm pressed from the plant
Colour: peach colour
Therapeutic properties: highly emollient, rich and nutritive. Contains essential fatty acids found in sebum
Skin types suitable for: all skin types, especially for dry and ageing skins

OLIVE OIL

KEY NOTE

This oil is very heavy and viscous, and tends to have a strong odour.

Botanical name: *Olea Europaea*
Source: extracted from hard, unripe olives
Colour: yellow-green

Therapeutic properties: rich and nutritive, contains a good source of vitamin E. Very soothing
Skin types suitable for: dehydrated skins and inflamed skin

PEACH KERNEL

KEY NOTE

This oil has a regenerative and tonic effect on the skin.

Botanical name: *Prunus persica*
Source: extracted from the kernel
Colour: pale green
Therapeutic properties: emollient, helps increase skin suppleness and elasticity. Contains vitamins A and E, and some essential fatty acids
Skin types suitable for: all skin types, especially dry and mature

SAFFLOWER

KEY NOTE

This oil is very economical to use as a carrier as it is inexpensive and light.

Botanical name: *Carthamux tinctorius*
Source: warm pressed from the seeds
Colour: yellow
Therapeutic properties: nutritive, as rich in essential fatty acids and vitamin E
Skin types suitable for: all skin types

ST JOHNS WORT

KEY NOTE

This oil is specially effective on healing wounds and soothing inflammation.

Botanical name: *Hypericum perforatum*
Source: macerated from the flowers and leaves
Colour: mauvey-red-brown

Therapeutic properties: anti-inflammatory, astringent, soothing and healing to the skin

Skin types suitable for: all skin types, especially dry and sensitive

SWEET ALMOND

> ### KEY NOTE
>
> This oil is probably one of the most popular carrier oils used in aromatherapy as it has a high therapeutic and nutritive value.

Botanical name: *Prunus amygdalus*

Source: warm pressed from the kernel of the sweet almond tree

Colour: pale yellow

Therapeutic properties: is soothing and calming and helps relieve itching. Contains vitamins A, B1, B2, B6, E and is rich in protein. Contains a high proportion of fatty acids

Skin types suitable for: all skin types, especially dry, ageing and inflamed skins.

SUNFLOWER

> ### KEY NOTE
>
> This oil is very fine and light and is a relatively neutral oil, making it effective for general purposes. It is relatively inexpensive.

Botanical name: *Helianthus annus*

Source: warm pressed from the sunflower seeds

Colour: golden yellow

Therapeutic properties: nutritive, contains fatty acids and high levels of vitamin E. Its structure is close to sebum

Skin types suitable for: all skin types, especially dry

WHEATGERM

> ### KEY NOTE
>
> This oil has a rich, viscous texture and is therefore too sticky to be used on its own. It is also highly odorous and if used to excess, will predominate the blend. Use up to 10% dilution with other carrier oils.

Botanical name: *Triticum vulgare*
Source: warm pressed from the germ of the wheat kernel
Colour: orange brown
Therapeutic properties: soothing, nourishing, healing. A natural anti-oxidant. A rich source of vitamin E and protein
Skin types suitable for: all skin types, especially inflamed and ageing

SUMMARY

KEY NOTE

- Carrier oils should be stored in a cold place for up to approximately nine months, after which time they will oxidise.
- As carrier oils are perishable products, it is wise to buy them frequently and in sensible proportions.
- When using carrier oils for therapeutic work, it is important to check that the client does not suffer from an allergy to nuts.

HOW TO BLEND OILS FOR AROMATHERAPY MASSAGE

The equipment needed to mix your essential oils will include the following:

- clear glass or plastic measuring container in mls
- selected essential oils
- selected carrier oils
- selection of dark glass bottles, ie 5 mls, 10 mls, 15 mls and 25 mls
- glass rod for stirring
- labels.

METHOD

- The amount of carrier/s required for the proposed treatment is measured out into the clear glass or plastic container, or measured directly into a dark glass bottle.
- The number of selected essential oil drops are then added one at a time, remembering to use a 2% dilution for the body and 1% for the face.
- If using a glass or plastic container, it is necessary to stir the mix with a glass rod or other suitable implement such as a spatula. If pouring into a bottle, the lid should be placed on the bottle and then shaken to disperse the essential oils into the carrier.

- If using a bottle, it is important to pour the oil up to the shoulder level of the bottle in order to leave an air gap.

> ————————— **KEY NOTE** —————————
>
> Always remember to label the blend if blending into bottles. If reusing the container and bottles, make sure that both are washed thoroughly and disinfected, to remove all trace of the previous blend of oils.

☞ TASK

Select a blend of oils for the following 'case histories' and state:
1 *which form of treatment you would be likely to use for this client;*
2 *the choice of essential oils and carrier oil/s used, along with the dilutions; and*
3 *what home care advice you would offer this client.*

- Miss S has cellulite and poor circulation. She also suffers with frequent headaches and has sensitive and dry skin.
- Mr N is an asthmatic with breathing difficulties. Also suffers with eczema and nervous tension. He has oily skin.
- Mrs D suffers extreme tension due to pressure of work, aches and muscular pains in the lumbar region of the back due to bending and lifting at work. Has normal skin, slightly dry.
- Mr J has mild hypertension and occasionally suffers with palpitations. He has just got over the breakdown of his marriage of 20 years and feels very inadequate. Has dry, sensitive skin.
- Miss K suffers with PMT and gets very irritable before a period, which is affecting her relationships at home. She also gets a lot of fluid retention and suffers with migraine. Has normal skin.
- Mrs Y has been taking tranquillisers for over 20 years, which were prescribed originally due to a nervous breakdown, following a bereavement of a close family member. She is very tense and complains of headaches and neck pain. Also has disturbing nightmares.

? SELF-ASSESSMENT QUESTIONS

1. What is meant by the term 'synergy' in aromatherapy?

   ....

   ....

   ....

   ....

2. State five important factors to be taken into account when blending essential oils.

   ....

   ....

   ....

   ....

   ....

3. What determines a choice of essential oils for a client in an aromatherapy treatment?

   ....

   ....

   ....

4. What determines the choice of carrier oil used for a client in aromatherapy?

   ....

   ....

5. List the therapeutic properties of the following carrier oils, indicating which skin type/s they may be suitable for:
   (i) Sweet almond

   ....

   ....

   ....

   ....

   ....

ii) Grapeseed

....

....

....

....

....

iii) Avocado

....

....

....

....

....

iv) Wheatgerm

....

....

....

....

....

v) Jojoba

....

....

....

....

....

Chapter 9

~

AROMATHERAPY MASSAGE AND OTHER FORMS OF TREATMENT

Aromatherapy massage represents the earliest form of treatment used in Roman and Egyptian times, and is still the primary form of treatment used in aromatherapy today. It allows the essential oils to absorb through the skin to affect the body and treats the body directly by the therapeutic effects of the massage itself.

- A competent aromatherapist needs to be able to prepare for and provide an aromatherapy massage incorporating a range of techniques.

By the end of this chapter you will be able to relate the following knowledge to your work as an aromatherapist:

- the range of aromatherapy massage techniques and their effects
- the hygiene and safety involved in preparing for an aromatherapy massage
- types of treatment given and commercial timings
- after-care advice given to a client following aromatherapy massage
- other forms of treatment using essential oils.

An aromatherapy massage has three main benefits:

- It aids absorption of essential oils into the bloodstream.
- There is the psychological benefit of inhaling the vapour itself.
- The massage itself has therapeutic effects and can relax and/or stimulate the client.

AROMATHERAPY MASSAGE TECHNIQUES

Massage is the most important method of application of aromatherapy, as it is the most effective way of introducing essential oils to affect the body systems, and there is the added benefit of therapeutic touch.

There is a wide variety in the massage techniques used by aromatherapists, depending on training and qualifications. However, aromatherapy massage techniques in general comprise of the Swedish massage techniques of *effleurage, petrissage, friction* and *vibrations*, alongside techniques such as *pressures* and *neuromuscular.* (See Mo Rosser, *Body Massage Therapy Basics*, 1996, Hodder & Stoughton, for a thorough explanation of massage techniques.)

Whatever method used, the movements used in aromatherapy are generally relaxing movements, omitting the more vigorous techniques such as *tapotement.* The movements are usually performed slowly, in order to induce relaxation and stress relief.

EFFLEURAGE

Technique

These are soothing and stroking movements which precede, connect and conclude any massage sequence. They are classified as *superficial* and *deep*.

Effleurage is performed with the palmar surface of the hand and should follow the venous and lymphatic flow. It is usually performed slowly as it is aimed at the slow circulation.

Effects

Effleurage:

- promotes venous flow, thereby increasing and improving general circulation
- increases lymphatic flow; hastens removal and absorption of waste products
- aids desquamation and increases the skin's elasticity
- improves the capillary circulation to the skin and nutrition to the skin's tissues
- provides continuity in the massage by linking other movements
- allow client to become accustomed to the aromatherapist's touch
- has a soothing effect on sensory nerve endings, inducing a state of relaxation
- aids oil absorption of essential oils into the bloodstream.

PETRISSAGE

Technique

This technique involves lifting the tissues away from the underlying structures and is often generically referred to as *kneading*. Pressure is smoothly and firmly applied and then relaxed. This movement should be performed with supple, relaxed hands which apply intermittent pressure with either one or both hands, or parts of the hands.

Effects

Petrissage:

- increases circulation and hastens elimination of waste from the tissues
- improves the tone and elasticity of muscles due to the increased blood supply
- aids relaxation of tense muscle fibres by carrying away products of fatigue and relieving pain.

FRICTIONS

Technique

These are small movements performed with the pad of the thumb or fingertips. They are small concentrated movements exerting controlled pressure on a small area of the surface tissues, moving them over the underlying structures.

Effects

Friction:

- stimulates circulation and metabolism within the tissues
- helps to break down and free skin adhesions
- aids absorption of fluid around joints
- presents the formation of fibrosis in the muscle tissue
- can have an invigorating or relaxing effect.

VIBRATIONS

Technique

These are fine trembling movements performed along a nerve path with one or both hands, using either the palmar surface of the hands or the fingertips.

Effects

Vibrations:

- stimulate and clear nerve pathways
- create a sedative effect, helping to relieve tension and refresh the client.

NEUROMUSCULAR

Technique

These are forms of massage techniques which use friction, vibration and pressure movements to help influence nerve pathways and muscles. They can help to release energy blocks by stimulating the nerves.

Effects

Neuromuscular techniques:

- stimulate the nerve supply to the corresponding organ
- stimulate cell renewal
- clear congestion in the nerves
- help to relieve muscular spasms.

PRESSURES

Technique

These techniques are performed by applying pressures on every inch of the skin with the thumbs or fingers, along the nerve tracts or meridians. These techniques are a form of 'energy' massage.

Effects

Pressures:

- stimulate the nerves and clear energy blocks
- ease congestion in the nervous system by relieving tension from the nerve tracts.

K E Y   N O T E

The increase in blood flow and warmth created by aromatherapy massage techniques increase the rate of absorption of essential oils into the bloodstream. Massage is therefore a very effective way of enhancing the absorption of oils to affect the systems of the body.

PREPARING FOR THE AROMATHERAPY MASSAGE

MAINTAINING EMPLOYMENT STANDARDS

An aromatherapist should present a smart and hygienic working appearance at all times, in order to project a professional attitude.

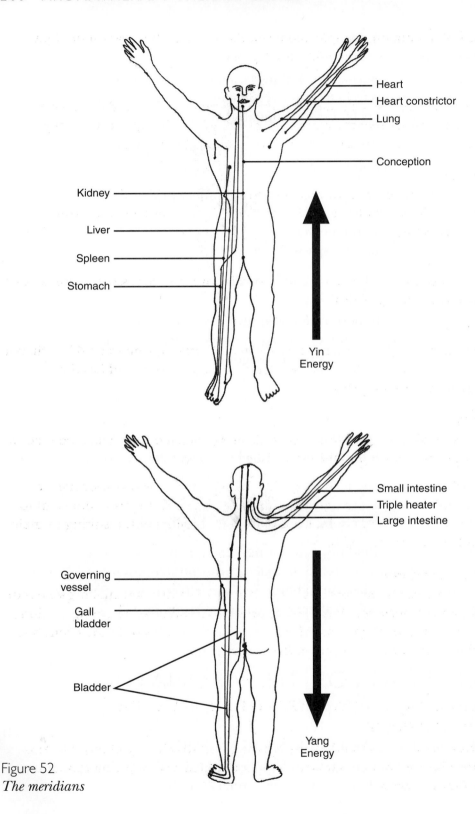

Heart
Heart constrictor
Lung

Conception

Kidney

Liver

Spleen

Stomach

Yin
Energy

Small intestine
Triple heater
Large intestine

Governing
vessel

Gall
bladder

Bladder

Yang
Energy

Figure 52
The meridians

As part of maintaining employment standards aromatherapists should pay particular attention to the following factors:

Clothing
Professional workwear should be worn at all times and should be clean and smart. Remember that the appearance of an aromatherapist can greatly influence a client into using their services on a regular basis.

Footwear
Footwear should be comfortable and clean, and matching the colour of workwear. Shoes should be flat or with a small heel, and enclosed (for hygiene reasons).

Hair
Long hair should be tied back with co-ordinating hair accessories; this is not only hygienic, but practical.

Jewellery
No jewellery should be worn for applying aromatherapy massage other than a wedding band, as jewellery may scratch or irritate a client and has the potential to harbour germs.

Hands
Hands should be kept as soft as possible and protected from harsh chemicals. Nails must be kept short and unvarnished.

Aromatherapists must ensure that they wash their hands very thoroughly before and after each treatment, for hygiene reasons. It is also important to ensure that they do not build up sensitivity to essential oils, resulting in their hands becoming cracked or sore.

Personal hygiene
Due to the close nature of working with aromatherapy, personal hygiene is of paramount importance. It is also important to avoid wearing strong smelling aftershaves and perfumes, as this may not only be offensive to the client but could interact with the aroma of the essential oils.

PREPARATION OF THE TREATMENT AREA FOR AROMATHERAPY
The treatment area should always look hygienically clean and tidy, but also comfortable and not too clinical. This can be achieved by giving thought to the following factors:

Lighting

This should be soft and discreet; try to avoid overhead lights which are glaring and not conducive to relaxation.

Ventilation

Ensure that the treatment area is well ventilated and draught free. It is advisable to air the room regularly between clients, by opening windows, to ensure the atmosphere remains fresh and that the build of aromas in the room is not too overpowering – this could make you or your client feel nauseous.

Temperature

This should be comfortably warm (approximately 70–75 degrees).

Decor and colours

Colouring should be chosen carefully as some colours are warm, whilst others will feel too cold and clinical. Towels should preferably match the decor and add to the warmth of the room.

Privacy

A treatment area should always be private to ensure client relaxation.

Atmosphere and noise level

Creating a relaxing atmosphere is a very important requirement of the aromatherapy massage, which can be aided by using a relaxation tape. Always ensure before you commence the aromatherapy massage, that you will not be disturbed by anyone entering the treatment room or a ringing phone.

HEALTH, SAFETY AND HYGIENE

As aromatherapy massage is a personalised treatment and there is close contact between the client and aromatherapist, there is a specific need to avoid cross-infection. In order to ensure health and safety, consideration should be given to:

- the treatment area and equipment used
- the client
- the aromatherapist.

THE TREATMENT AREA

In order to adhere to all health, safety and hygiene requirements, attention must be paid to the following:

- keep the treatment area hygienically clean at all times

- keep the area free from obstructions
- ensure that all equipment is regularly disinfected
- ensure all floor coverings are slip-proof
- install hand washing facilities in the vicinity of the treatment area
- dispose of all rubbish in a lined and covered bin; empty at regular intervals
- check all equipment is stable and fit for use by checking all hinges and locks
- maintain all electrical equipment regularly by having it checked by a qualified engineer once a year
- be familiar with the location and the correct usage of fire extinguishers
- clearly indicate all fire exits and fire evacuation procedures
- keep a well-maintained first aid kit in the treatment area
- store all product equipment correctly and safely
- ensure the correct maintenance of heating and ventilation systems.

THE CLIENT

- check client for contra-indications to ensure they are suitable for treatment
- use clean towels and disposable tissue covering, for each client
- wash hands before and after each client to avoid cross-infection
- check the client for any contagious or infectious disorders
- ensure client has removed all jewellery
- avoid open wounds and sores and ensure they are covered with a waterproof plaster
- do not give an aromatherapy massage if you are ill or contagious
- check client's skin type before treatment; if necessary, do a skin test to avoid skin irritation and sensitisation resulting from the incorrect use of essential oils
- help clients on and off the massage couch
- ensure client is hygienically prepared for treatment by showering to remove all perfumes and cosmetics, wearing a suitable head covering if hair is long and that they retain their pants.

THE AROMATHERAPIST

- present a smart and hygienic appearance at all times
- always wear professional workwear
- cover all cuts or abrasions with a waterproof plaster
- avoid cross infection by using disposable spatulas to remove any products; keep lids tightly on bottles
- use correctly lifting techniques when moving equipment
- use correct posture and stance when carrying out aromatherapy massage

- use equipment and products in accordance with manufacturer's instructions
- wash hands thoroughly before and after each client
- maintain first aid skills
- know the location of the first aid kit and fire evacuation procedures
- be familiar with the fire fighting equipment
- be familiar with contra-indications so as to know when a client may be treated and when they should be referred to a medical practitioner.

AROMATHERAPY MASSAGE PROCEDURE

There are three main forms of treatment offered in aromatherapy massage. The choice will depend on the client's needs and preference, and most probably the cost.

- Full aromatherapy massage – usually takes between 1 hour, and 1 hour and 15 minutes
- Full aromatherapy massage including the face and scalp – usually takes 1 hour and a half
- Part body aromatherapy massage applied locally to body parts – usually takes between 30 and 45 minutes, depending on which areas are treated.

── KEY NOTE ──

Whatever method of treatment is given, it is essential that it is adapted to suit the individual needs of the client. A client's needs will vary from treatment to treatment, and there may be a need to change the previous treatment plan due to a change in the client's condition or circumstances.

It is also important to ensure that the treatment given is cost-effective in terms of time.

BEFORE THE MASSAGE

Follow these guidelines to ensure a safe and effective aromatherapy massage:

- Carry out a consultation to identify whether the client is unsuitable for treatment, and check for contra-indications.
- Complete records; check that the client agrees with the information and signs the declaration.
- Assess client needs to establish the objectives of the treatment.

- Formulate a treatment plan with the client: the treatment objectives, the treatment method and the time it will take.
- Select and blend oils ready for use, and ask client to approve the selection.
- Check that all necessary working materials are to hand and the treatment area and couch have been correctly prepared with clean towels and tissues.
- Advise the client to empty their bladder and disrobe ready for treatment.
- Ensure client is warm, comfortable and relaxed before treatment commences.

KEY NOTE

If the face and scalp is to be included in the treatment, you will need to ensure that the client's face has been cleansed and is free from cosmetics and make-up before treatment.

AFTER-CARE ADVICE

The following advice should be given to a client following aromatherapy massage:

- **Avoid skin washing and bathing** for approximately eight hours after treatment as this will enable the essential oils to fully penetrate the skin and have their effects on the body through the bloodstream. Most essential oils can take up to 60 minutes to absorb through the skin and can carry out their therapeutic work for up to 8 hours afterwards.
- **Avoid direct exposure to strong sunlight** following the use of any phototoxic oils.
- **Avoid alcohol and smoking:** it is important for a client not to smoke or drink for at least 24 hours after treatment as aromatherapy massage is a detoxifying treatment.
- **Drink plenty of fresh water and herbal infusions:** as aromatherapy is essentially a cleansing treatment, drinking plenty of water and herbal teas can assist in the elimination of toxins from the body and help the healing process.
- **Eat a light diet:** it is important to eat a light and natural diet as the body needs to concentrate its effort on detoxification and natural healing. Fresh and natural foods are advisable, because over-refined and processed food adds to the toxicity of the body.
- **Enjoy rest and relaxation:** in order to assist the healing process, the client should be advised to rest as much as possible following treatment. Clients will invariably feel tired after treatment and they will benefit from a good rest. The feeling of tiredness will often be replaced by a feeling of vitality.

POST-AROMATHERAPY MASSAGE PROCEDURE

- allow the client to rest while you wash your hands thoroughly to remove all residue of oils
- offer client a glass of water
- allow client to change and help them off the couch
- offer client after-care advice
- evaluate the effectiveness of the treatment by gaining feedback from the client. Ask how they are feeling and whether treatment has been successful in meeting the overall treatment objectives
- review the treatment plan with the client
- make recommendations for a future treatment and book the client's next appointment
- complete treatment records ensuring that you have kept an accurate record of essential oils used, dates and results.

——— K E Y   N O T E ———

In order to enhance the effects of the massage, aromatherapists may wish to make up individual bath oils for clients to use at home. Remember that all blends given to clients must be clearly labelled, with their contents, amounts used and the date blended. It is also advisable to include an expiry date.

☞ TASK

In order to gain as much experience in aromatherapy as possible, carry out several case studies which will involve many clients having aromatherapy massage treatments over a period of time.

Try to select as wide a range of clients as possible both in terms of age and condition. After undertaking a full consultation with them:

- formulate and agree a treatment plan
- perform aromatherapy massage techniques over a period of time, using a range of aromatherapy massage movements
- evaluate the effectiveness of the treatments
- advise the client on after care and home care procedures.

OTHER FORMS OF TREATMENT

Although massage should always be the primary form of treatment, there are instances when massage may be inappropriate or when other forms of treatments may be used to enhance the effectiveness of treatment.

AROMATIC BATHS

This method is useful for client's self-use and may be used between treatments to reinforce the treatment given by the aromatherapist.

Method

Essential oils may be added directly to the bath water or blended in carrier oil first. If adding the essential oils directly to the water, take care to disperse in the water as the oils will not dilute in the water, but will float on the top.

A safe amount of essential oil to add to the bath to use is up to **six** drops of most oils. *Note:* Oils such as *lemon* and *peppermint* need to be restricted to **two** or **three** drops only, as they could cause adverse skin reactions if used to excess. There are certain essential oils such as *clove* and *cinnamon* which are unsuitable for use in the bath as they are skin irritants.

KEY NOTE

Never use undiluted oils in the bath for babies, young children and those with sensitive skin: always dilute them in a carrier oil first.

If making up an aromatic bath oil for a client, the same dilution rate of 2% essential oil to carrier oil applies. Always ensure you have labelled the blend and that you have instructed the client on self use. Usually one or two capfuls will be sufficient for a bath with the recommended treatment time of 15–20 minutes.

HAND AND FOOT BATHS

These can be useful to treat areas which cannot be massaged, for example an arthritic or otherwise injured limb.

Method

The amount of essential oils would be restricted to two–four drops for a hand bath and two–six drops for a foot bath, depending on the choice of oils.

The hands and feet are highly penetrative areas and if someone cannot be obviously treated with massage, then it is a useful way of absorbing the oils into the bloodstream for therapeutic benefit.

STEAM INHALATION

This method is especially suited to sinus, throat and chest infections.

Method

A single drop may be enough, and four drops is the maximum. Try one drop only the first time: **do not inhale for longer than about 60 seconds at a time if you have a history of asthma or allergies**.

Provided this is well tolerated, you can then increase the amount of oil used and lengthen the treatment time to five minutes or more.

COMPRESSES

This is a very effective way of using essential oils to relieve pain and reduce inflammation.

Method

A *hot compress* may be made by filling a bowl with very hot water and then adding four or five drops of essential oil (depending on the oil). Dip a piece of absorbent material such as cotton wool or a flannel or lint into the water, squeeze out the excess and then place over the affected area until it is has cooled, then repeat. Hot compresses are particularly useful for backache, earache, rheumatism, arthritis, abscesses, earache and toothache.

Cold compresses are made in a similar way, using ice cold rather than hot water and these are useful for headaches, sprains, strains and hot, swollen conditions.

BURNERS AND VAPORISERS

This method is used for vaporising essential oils in a room. The simplest form of *burner* involves a night light and a section which is filled with water.

Method

Up to 12 drops of essential oil may be added to the water section of the burner. The heat of the night light evaporates the water and the essential oil, vaporising the odour into the atmosphere.

Another way of diffusing essential oils into the atmosphere involves a small heating element and a small pad onto which the drops of essential oil are placed – this is more commonly known as a *vaporiser*.

─────────── **KEY NOTE** ───────────

Great care must be taken when using burners to ensure that they do not get knocked over and that they are not placed near flammable materials.

BLENDING WITH CREAMS

Essential oils may be blended into base creams for client self application, as the client may find it easier and more convenient to apply a cream or lotion as part of their home care treatment.

Method

- Take an unperfumed cream or lotion.
- Add any special carriers to the cream/lotion first, a little at a time and mix well.
- Fill the pot or jar with three-quarters of the required cream/lotion and then add the essential oils and shake well.
- Add the rest of the cream/lotion and leave a 10% air gap to ensure an even blend of oils.
- Label and ensure you have given the client clear instruction for self application.

─────────── **KEY NOTE** ───────────

It is recommended that the blending ratio for cream and lotions is between 1–5%, depending on the reasons for usage.

Base creams or lotions may be bought from good essential oil suppliers. They should be unperfumed and made from pure and natural plant substances.

? SELF-ASSESSMENT QUESTIONS

I. Why is massage one of the most effective ways of absorbing essential oils into the bloodstream for therapeutic effect?

....

....

....

....

2. Describe the effects of the following movements used in aromatherapy massage:
   i) effleurage

....

....

....

....

....

....

   ii) neuromuscular

....

....

....

....

....

   iii) pressures

....

....

....

....

3. State five important health and safety factors when preparing the treatment area for an aromatherapy massage.

....

....

....

....

....

....

4. State five important health and safety factors when preparing the client for aromatherapy massage.

....

....

....

....

....

....

5. What general after-care advice should be offered to a client following an aromatherapy massage and why?

....

....

....

....

....

....

....

....

....

....

....

....

Chapter 10

BASIC BUSINESS SKILLS FOR THE AROMATHERAPIST

As complementary therapies continue to grow in popularity, more and more business opportunities are developing which will enable therapists to practise aromatherapy professionally.

Whether self-employed, managing a business, or working as an employee, it is very important to be able to understand *and* implement good business practice.

- A competent aromatherapist needs to be able to understand the principles of business management in order to be successful and ensure the smooth running of a business.

By the end of this chapter you will be able to relate the following to your work as an aromatherapist:

- the requirements for setting up an aromatherapy practice
- marketing and advertising
- professional ethics
- professional associations.

In order to run a successful aromatherapy practice, it is important not only to be good at the skill you practise but also to develop good business skills which will help you to maintain *and* develop your business.

Being a good aromatherapist is not enough to ensure a successful business. One of the main reasons that small businesses fail at an early stage is due to poor management.

A successful business depends on

- a good image
- a good reputation
- a high degree of professionalism
- sufficient resources to deliver a quality service
- effective record keeping.

MAINTAINING EMPLOYMENT STANDARDS

There are several important factors to take account of when working as an aromatherapist in order to maintain and monitor the standard of service you offer to clients.

It is not only important to perform a skill competently but to be able to apply it in a commercially acceptable way.

Aromatherapists must bear in mind at all times that they are part of the service industry, and the following factors could affect the day-to-day running and the overall efficiency of the business:

- communication skills
- management and staff responsibilities
- working conditions
- establishment rules and quality assurance
- record keeping
- resources – planning and monitoring.

COMMUNICATION SKILLS

Whether a sole trader or a large business, a successful business relies on good communication. Communication skills are extremely important when there are several colleagues working together in the same clinic, and information needs to be conveyed and received.

If communication skills are broken down for as little as half an hour in a busy clinic, it can have a very dramatic effect on the service given and the overall efficiency and image of the clinic. Good communication means being able to liaise well with clients, colleagues and other visitors who may enter or telephone the clinic, such as a supplier or another fellow professional.

Communication may involve:

- talking
- listening

- writing
- eye contact
- body language.

When communicating with clients or colleagues over the telephone or in person, it is very important to have good *listening* skills, to ensure that you have received the information they are trying to convey to you correctly.

It is very important to *clarify* what a client has said before acting on it, to ensure that you have received the right information. It is equally important that when you are speaking to a client or a colleague, that you *speak clearly* and accurately to ensure that everything has been understood.

It is most important that *non-verbal* signs that you send out reflect what you are saying. Non-verbal signs are usually picked up from posture, facial expressions and gestures. Try to use effective *body language*, so that you appear friendly and approachable, even when you are not speaking.

Eye contact is very important when talking and listening. Remember that your personal presentation will make a lasting impression, and so you should project a professional image from the start.

Written communication

Recording information accurately is very important for communication, particularly when colleagues are very busy with clients and do not have much face-to-face contact with other colleagues.

Communication should be up-to date, easily understood and in a place where the person is likely to see it and take notice of it.

Messages should include a time, date and the action required, along with the caller's name and a contact number, if it is an external enquiry.

Written communication also includes effective record keeping; see page 117.

MANAGEMENT RESPONSIBILITIES

When working in a clinic or alongside other professionals, it is very important to know your colleagues' responsibilities as well as your own, to ensure a smooth operation of quality service to clients.

☞ TASK I

Below is a list of the usual hierarchy in a team of professionals (not all of them would apply to a small clinic). Write what you feel their individual responsibilities should be in each case.

Draw a flow chart to show the order of command. This may be entered into your portfolio for evidence collection.

Proprietor

....

....

....

....

....

Line Manager/Supervisor

....

....

....

....

....

Therapist

....

....

....

....

....

Receptionist

....

....

....

....

....

WORK CONDITIONS

Work conditions should ensure maximum satisfaction to both clients and staff, and is dependent on the following factors:

- the working environment (heating, lighting, ventilation)
- equipment and materials (sufficient in quality and quantity to carry out work to a client's satisfaction and in a commercially acceptable time)
- procedures – these are set by the management; all staff should be aware of the necessary work procedures to enhance smooth running of the clinic.

ESTABLISHMENT RULES

Work activities in a clinic must comply with:

- the individual establishment's rules
- legislation and the industry's Code of Practice (ie hygiene, health and safety)
- customer requirements.

Every establishment should therefore have a set of 'house rules' so that the employees know what is required of them at the beginning of each day, throughout the course of the day and at the end of each day.

◐ TASK 2

Draw up a list of clinic manager's duties, including establishment rules and policies.

QUALITY ASSURANCE

Most companies or businesses, however small, should have a quality assurance policy to ensure that their business is conducted in a systematic way. A quality assurance policy:

- will ensure that customer needs and improvements for quality are met, and that they are reviewed regularly
- monitors the quality and standard of the service, and the cost-effectiveness and viability of the business
- is set to ensure that the service delivers exactly what the providers claim it does, and does so consistently; quality is all about 'fitness for purpose'
- is a useful and essential part of planning in a business, as it identifies client needs and ensures that the aims of the business and customer needs are met efficiently, effectively and consistently.

RECORD KEEPING

An efficient clinic relies on accurate, legible record keeping, which is kept up-to-date and may be either hand-written or computer-based. Record keeping includes keeping accurate client records, stock records and any other records of importance such as an accident book.

An important factor to remember with client records is to maintain client confidentiality. All records should be kept in a secure environment, and a client's personal details should never be left lying around for anyone to read.

Stock records and simple accounts records are an essential part of the day-to-day running of the business. They should be done regularly so that you may keep a control on the financial resources of the business.

RESOURCES

Resources are the means by which you conduct your business. Resources must be **planned**, **monitored** and **controlled** to ensure that you stay in business. The planning, monitoring and controlling of resources involves a combination of the following:

Staff

Adequate staff resources are essential to a successful business. The optimum situation is to have the maximum staff available at the busy times and the minimum in the quiet times. Staff costs money and their time must be used efficiently. If they are not earning money for the business, consideration must be given to what they can do in the quiet times to promote business.

Information

Planning and monitoring resources involves good communication between clients and colleagues. It is essential that staff are aware of resources, and how they can be controlled by minimising waste and being cost-effective. Staff may also contribute to the planning by indicating to the manager/manageress that stock is low and needs to be reordered, or even suggesting a new supplier who is more efficient and economical.

Staff must also be well informed about treatments available in the clinic, so that they can provide information to prospective clients and sell the service effectively.

Materials

This involves all items of stock and consumables used in the clinic. An accurate record should be kept of all stock in the clinic in a stock control book. Stock records are essential, to ensure that there is adequate stock at all times and to avoid being faced with a disappointed client if you find that you do not have the materials to do the job.

It is equally important not to be over-stocked, as you will be tying up any available capital and stock will deteriorate with age.

Stock control should ideally be carried out on a weekly basis.

TASK 3

Design a simple stock record sheet which may be utilised to carry out a stock check in the clinic

Equipment

These are the tools required to perform the treatments you offer. Equipment should be regularly checked and serviced and a record should be kept of this.

Treatments must be planned to ensure cost-effectiveness, taking account of *money, time* and *services.*

FINANCE

Controlling finance is essential to an efficient business. A daily cash book is important, as this keeps a daily record of all financial transactions.

It is vital to keep a close eye on your account and your profit margin, and to look at ways in which you can save money, without cutting down on quality.

You will need to have a short-term and/or long-term financial plan. Short-term planning may involve an overdraft to get you out of a difficult patch, and for the long term you may require a loan to accommodate future plans.

TIME

Timing is an essential factor to consider, so that you:

- avoid keeping other clients waiting
- minimise potential inconvenience to a client
- ensure a cost-effective treatment.

SERVICES

These are the services or treatments you offer to a client in the clinic which must be accurate in terms of information provided, and take account of consumer legislation, as well as customer requirements.

BUSINESS PLANNING

Running a successful business involves an incredible amount of planning. In the long term, the time spent planning will help to create more business and save you from wasting valuable money, time and resources.

No matter how efficient or successful a business, every service can be improved, even if only in a small way; every business should involve short term and long term planning.

RESEARCH PLAN

Formulating a research plan is essential when considering starting your own business as it enables you to assess the *potential* of the project, along with its costs and estimated income. There are certain costs associated with a new business, which may include the following:

- rent or lease
- utilities (electricity, lighting)
- equipment and supplies
- furniture
- decorating
- stationery and printing
- advertising
- insurance
- legal and professional fees.

There are many factors to consider when formulating a research plan:

Client requirements

- Decide what client market you are aiming at and the individual needs of those clients.
- Ask yourself whether their needs will be met by your service and available resources.
- Carry out some market research by formulating surveys and questionnaires, to assess the need for your service in your area.

Premises

Decide whether to work from home or from a commercial premises (leasehold or freehold); state the advantages and disadvantages of both.

Catchment area

Look into the catchment area and decide who your potential customers are. You may also wish to consider the competition in your catchment area, and how your service will differ from theirs.

Specialist advice

Consider what professional help you will need in setting up your business, and perhaps enlist the help of a business advisor, accountant or solicitor.

Legal requirements

Consider what legal requirements you will need to take account of to ensure good commercial practice, and what legislation (local and national) is relevant to your business.

Finance

What finance do you have available, to inject into the business? Will it be self-financed or externally financed? Look at the advantages and disadvantages of short-term (overdrafts) and long-term finance (loans).

Equipment

What equipment and materials will you need to carry out the plan, and how much will it all cost? What stock will you need and in what quantity? Make a list of all expenditure, so that you may assess the starting-up costs.

☞ TASK 4

Imagine you are planning to start your own business, either from home or from commercial premises. You might be starting or improving an existing business, by adding an additional skill to the business, for example.

Prepare a research plan in outline, taking account of the factors above.

OPERATIONAL PLAN

An operational plan is the next stage from the research plan as it sets out the actual *running* of the business.

You will need to take account of the following:

- **What services do you intend to offer?** Draw up a price list which includes a detailed description of the treatments on offer, the price and the time allocated to each treatment.
- **Which hours of business do you intend to operate?** Consider what times clients will be available to use your services, in order to maximise your business opportunity.
- **What price do you intend to charge for the services?** The prices you charge will be dependent on the market, competition, catchment area and your individual overheads. Remember that the service you offer is unique to you and therefore you must value it first in order to put a price on your

service. Consider how much you intend to earn and what the potential income of the business is, by considering the income against the expenditure.

- **What staff will you need and at what times?** If you are a sole trader, you may just require an answer-phone to take your messages when you are busy with clients, or you may wish to employ a receptionist to book your appointments.
- **How do you intend to advertise your services?** Consider the different ways in which you can inform clients of your services.
- **What can you do to ensure good public relations and a good professional image?** Consider the ways in which you can project a good public image through your business.
- **How will you ensure quality assurance?** Consider how you can improve on customer service and enhance client satisfaction.
- **What will you need to protect your business interests?** Consider the types of insurance required for your business in the event of any loss. Comply with any legal or professional association requirements.

MARKETING

The aim of marketing is to *promote* and *increase* your business, and is the means by which you inform clients of your services.

As aromatherapy is a very personal service, you will need to target your market to specific client groups in order to get effective results. First of all, you need to decide which client market you want to attract, and then you must direct your marketing at them.

With a new business, you need to spend time on making contacts; this may involve giving talks and presentations on aromatherapy and how it can benefit your potential clients. Networking with other professionals (such as physiotherapists, GPs, homeopaths, hypnotherapists) can be another useful way of marketing your services. You can inform them of your services in writing; if you obtain information from them, you may promote referrals between you, in an effort to facilitate a holistic health care approach.

PROMOTION

Design attractive and informative promotional material which may be targeted at specific client groups; for example, if you wish to attract clients at a local health club, then inquire if you can display one of your leaflets on their notice board. Remember that promotional material must be eye-catching and not too wordy. In general, potential clients will want to know four main things when considering using your service:

- How much will it cost?
- How long does it take?
- Why should I use the service, ie what are its benefits?
- Where is the service provided and at what times?

When designing promotional materials, sell the benefits of your service rather than a lengthy description of what it is, and try to identify with your client group in order to personalise the marketing.

If you have an existing business, concentrate on targeting your existing clients by writing to them to inform them of your newly acquired skill and how it could help them.

In order to create more new business from your clientele, you may wish to reward existing clients with an incentive scheme to introduce new clients into your business.

Remember that regular, satisfied clients are the most valuable asset to a business – by ensuring that you keep your clients happy, you are maintaining your quality assurance.

ADVERTISING

There are various forms of advertising to promote your business, but these need to be budgeted for carefully, and evaluated regularly for their effectiveness. A simple way of evaluating the effectiveness of your advertising is to ask each new enquiry you receive how they heard of you; this will enable you to discover which advertising is working for you.

There are several forms of advertising which involve cost, and these include:

- newspaper advertising
- national directories
- exhibitions
- promotional literature.

Newspaper advertising, display or classified

This form of advertising can be expensive (particularly display advertising), and its effectiveness can be dependent on the page the advert appears on and the day it is being delivered. Newspapers have a very short life span and therefore your message in the advert needs to be fairly dramatic to command attention from a wider audience. You will also need to advertise frequently to make the advertising effective.

National directories

National directories such as 'Yellow Pages', are produced once a year and are a more targeted form of advertising as there is a classification for services such as aromatherapy. This means that your advertising will be targeted at those who choose to look up your services.

Exhibitions

These are an effective way of marketing your services to a target audience, and although time-consuming, the actual costs involved will be minimal. It also gives you a means to communicate directly with your potential clients and affords you the opportunity to demonstrate your skills to a target audience.

Promotional literature (leaflets and mailshots)

These may be targeted at specific client groups and may include special offers or the introduction of a new service. Promotional literature may be dropped into the doors of a particular catchment area or placed in several prominent places within the community (notice boards at schools, universities, hospitals etc.).

The most effective forms of advertising are usually free. For example:

- **Word of mouth**   if you work hard to keep your existing clients happy, they will willingly market your services for you by telling their friends and colleagues.
- **Talks and demonstrations**   giving a talk to a particular client group is an ideal way of communicating the benefits of your service to a target audience. It is a good form of public relations which gives you the opportunity to present a positive public image.
- Always take some promotional materials and business cards to give out to the group you are talking or demonstrating to, so that they may read about its benefits and know where to contact you for an appointment.

An essential aspect of business development is good *public relations.* Networking with other professionals and developing personal and professional contacts are good ways of giving and receiving support as well as sharing resources and information.

Contact your local enterprise agency and chamber of commerce – if you become a member, this will open out new contacts for you in business.

PROFESSIONAL ETHICS

Professional ethics are standards of acceptable professional behaviour by which a person or business conducts their business. Each professional association has its own code of ethics to which members must adhere.

The following guidelines reflect, in general terms, a code of ethics expected in the aromatherapy industry. A professional aromatherapist must:

- not treat any person who is suffering from a medical condition; if a client presents a medical condition, s/he should be referred to the GP
- conduct themselves in a professional manner and be courteous and respectful to a client at all times
- always bear in mind that their primary concern should be for the client and that they should practise their skills to the best of their ability at all times
- have respect for the religious, spiritual, social or political views of the clients, irrespective of creed, race, colour or sex
- never abuse the relationship between themselves and a client
- act in a co-operative manner with other health care professionals and refer cases which are out of the sphere of the therapy field in which they practise
- explain the treatment and discuss any fees involved with the client before any treatment commences
- keep accurate, up-to-date records of treatments carried out on a client and the results; these records should include client's confidential details, a medical history, dates and details of treatment and any advice given
- never disclose client information without the prior written permission of the client, except when required to do so by law
- never claim to cure
- never diagnose a medical condition
- never give unqualified advice
- keep their personal and professional life separate
- ensure that any advertising represents their business in the most professional manner
- ensure that their working premises comply with all current health, safety and hygiene legislation
- be adequately insured to practise the therapy in which they are qualified
- become a member of a professional association who sets high standards for the industry
- continue their own professional development.

PROFESSIONAL ASSOCIATIONS

Becoming a member of a professional association helps to give you an identity as a professional and has many other benefits, including:

- a badge and certificate to display to the public which reflects the trademark of a professional

- professional indemnity insurance at a very reasonable rate, which is negotiated by your professional association
- regular magazines and newsletters which keep you up-to-date with the latest information on the industry
- an advisory service
- regular meetings and seminars to meet other colleagues and update your knowledge.

INSURANCE

Insurance is a necessity in business as it helps to protect your assets. Listed below are different types of insurance:

- **Professional indemnity** this protects you in the event of a claim arising from malpractice.
- **Public liability** this protects you in the case of a client or member of public becoming injured on your premises.
- **Employer's liability** this is a legal requirement if you employ staff. It protects an employer against any claims brought about by an employee who may get injured on the premises. A certificate of employer's liability must be displayed in the clinic.
- **Product liability** this type of insurance protects you against claims arising from products used. In the case of aromatherapy, if you are making up blends for client's self-use, it is essential for you to have 'selling-on liability'.
- **Buildings insurance** this protects the building against damage such as fire, explosion, flood or storm damage, accidental damage etc. If you are working from home, review your household policy concerning the liability of operating a business from home. If you are renting, it will usually be the landlord's responsibility to insure the building against the perils listed above. Ask for a copy of the policy to check that it is current.
- **Contents insurance** this protects your stock, equipment and fittings in your clinic against damage or loss.
- **Personal accident insurance** this protects you against loss of income in the event of an accident preventing you from working. Policies of this nature have certain exclusions and restrictions, and advice should be sought from your professional association or through a broker to ensure that you obtain the best policy.

REGULATING HEALTH AND SAFETY IN THE WORKPLACE

An important part of being an aromatherapist and running a clinic is understanding and following health, safety and hygiene regulations to develop safe working practises.

In order to ensure a healthy, safe and secure working environment for yourself, clients and colleagues, it is essential for the aromatherapist to be familiar with the implications of the following legislation and information:

1 **The Industry Code of Practice for Hygiene in Beauty Salons and Clinics** (published by Vocational Training Charitable Trust). This specifies correct hygiene precautions in order to avoid cross-infection.

2 Legislation relating to **hygiene** and **safety**, including:

- Local Government Miscellaneous Provisions Act 1982
- Local authority bye-laws
- The Health and Safety At Work Act 1974 (procedures in the event of accidents, spillages, breakages)
- First Aid at work
- Fire Precautions Act 1971 (fire and emergency procedures)
- The Control of Substances Hazardous To Health Regulations 1994, COSHH

3 **Consumer protection** legislation, including:

- Sales of Goods Act 1979
- Consumer Protection Act 1987
- Trade Descriptions Act 1968

LEGISLATION RELATING TO HEALTH AND SAFETY

Health, safety and hygiene is of paramount importance in the workplace. The Law requires that every place of employment is a healthy and safe place, not only for those employees who work there, but also for clients and other visitors who may enter the workplace.

Local Government (Miscellaneous Provisions) Act 1982; Local authority bye-laws

The primary concern of this Act is with efficient hygienic practice.

Bye-laws vary between local authorities, as does the licensing and inspection system involved. Bye-laws are made by the local authority to ensure:

- the cleanliness of the premises and fittings
- the cleanliness and hygiene of the persons registered, and their assistants
- the sterilisation and disinfection of instruments, materials and equipment used.

Large local authorities may have their own legislation under which similar establishments to beauty salons are licensed. In such cases, the licensing may cover what are termed 'special treatments', and this usually includes massage and the provision of ultra-violet treatments. In some areas, saunas are licensed and in others not.

It is wise to seek the advice of your local authority Environmental Health Officer regarding local legislation which may affect your business.

In areas where licensing and registration is required, it is important to remember that those working from home or those undertaking home visiting are still required to register. Only operators working under medical control (as in a hospital) are specifically excluded from registration.

Note: *Local Environmental Officers have the authority to fine or cancel the registration of a business which does not maintain and monitor safe hygienic practices.*

The Health and Safety at Work Act 1974

The Health and Safety at Work Act 1974 provides a comprehensive legal framework to promote and encourage high standards of health and safety in the workplace. Under this Act, everyone working in a clinic or salon is obliged to follow all safety guidelines and to have consideration for their fellow workers.

Both employer and employee have responsibilities under this Act:

The *Employer* must:

- safeguard as far as possible the health, safety and welfare of themselves, their employees, contractor's employees and members of the public
- keep all equipment up to standard
- have safety equipment checked regularly
- ensure the environment is free from toxic fumes
- ensure all staff are aware of safety procedures, by providing safety information and training
- ensure safe systems of work.

The *Employee* must:

- take reasonable care to avoid injury to themselves and others
- co-operate with others

- not interfere or wilfully misuse anything provided to protect their health and safety.

Note: *The Health and Safety Executive have produced a guide to the laws on Health and Safety and it is a legal requirement that an employer displays a copy of this poster at a place of work.*

Fire Precautions Act 1971

This Act enforces that:

- all premises have fire fighting equipment which is in good working order
- the equipment is readily available and suitable for the types of fire that are likely to occur (A Carbon Dioxide gas (black) and dry powder extinguisher (blue) would be most suitable for salon/clinic use.)
- doors are left unlocked and that a quick exit can be made in the event of a fire
- room contents do not obstruct exits.

The responsibilities of an employee are to:

- keep flammable products away from heat
- avoid overloading electrical circuits
- avoid trailing electric leads, where they can be tripped over
- switch off and unplug all electrical appliances after use
- not smoke in the building
- avoid placing towels over electric or gas heaters.

✏ TASK 5

Check the health and safety regulations in your college or clinic. What is the procedure in the event of a fire or an accident?

Control of Substances Hazardous to Health 1994, COSHH

This Act requires employers to control people's exposure to hazardous substances in the workplace. Some products used in a clinic are safe in normal circumstances, but can become hazardous in certain conditions; for example, essential oils are highly flammable if exposed to naked flames.

Note: *always read the manufacturer's instructions relating to the use and storage of products and substances.*

CONSUMER LEGISLATION

It is important for a therapist to be aware of consumer legislation, in the unfortunate event of dealing with an unhappy client who is seeking compensation for products or services received.

Consumer Protection Act 1987

In the past, injured persons had to prove that a manufacture was negligent, before they could successfully sue for damages. The Consumer Protection Act 1987 removed this need to prove negligence. A customer can already sue a supplier without proof of negligence under the Sale of Goods Act 1976, but the Consumer Protection Act 1987 provides the same rights to anyone injured by a defective product, whether the product was sold to them or not.

This Act also covers the giving of misleading price indications about goods, services or facilities (the term 'price indication' also includes price comparisons). To be misleading includes any wrongful indications about conditions attached to a price, what you expect to happen to a price in the future and what you say in price comparisons. As an offence could result in criminal proceedings, it is essential that there is a good understanding of what is involved, even in relation to special offers.

Sale of Goods Act 1979/The Supply of Goods and Services Act 1982

As consumers of products and services, clients have rights under the Sale of Goods Act 1982 and the Supply of Goods and Services Act 1982.

This legislation identifies the contract of sale which takes place between the retailer (the clinic) and the consumer (the client). They cover consumer rights, including ensuring that goods are of merchandable quality, the conditions under which goods may be returned after purchase and whether goods are fit for their intended purpose.

A client disappointed with a treatment could take action against the clinic if it was proved that reasonable care had not been taken under the terms of the Supply of Goods and Services Act 1982.

Trade Descriptions Act 1968

This Act prohibits the use of false descriptions to sell or offer the sale of goods. It covers advertisements such as oral descriptions, and display cards, and applies to quality and quantity as well as fitness for purpose and price.

Note: you will break this law even if you are repeating a description given by another person; therefore to repeat a manufacturer's claim is to be equally liable.

? SELF-ASSESSMENT QUESTIONS

1. What are the responsibilities of an employer under the Health and Safety at Work Act 1974?

....

....

....

....

....

....

2. State four requirements of the Fire Precautions Act 1971.

....

....

....

....

....

3. Explain what is meant by the legislation entitled COSHH.

....

....

....

4. What is the importance of adhering to consumer legislation as a practising aromatherapist?

....

....

5. State five important types of insurance requirements when practising as an aromatherapist.

....

....

....

....

....

....

6. Why are professional ethics important to a practising aromatherapist?

....

....

....

BIBLIOGRAPHY

Berwick, Ann (1994) *Holistic Aromatherapy*, Llewellyn Publication

Bettelheim & March (1990) *Introduction to Organic Biochemistry*

Davis, Patricia (1995) *Aromatherapy, an A–Z*, C.W. Daniel Company Ltd

Lawless, Julia (1995) *The Illustrated Encyclopaedia of Essential Oils*, Elements Books

Price, Shirley (1993) *Shirley Price's Aromatherapy Workbook*, Thorsons

Price, Shirley and Len (1995) *Aromatherapy for Health Professionals*, Churchill Livingstone.

Rosser, Mo (1996) *Body Massage Therapy Basics*, Hodder & Stoughton

Skoog, West & Holler (1992) *Fundamentals of Analytical Chemistry*

Tisserand, Robert (1991) *The Art of Aromatherapy*, C.W. Daniel Company Ltd

Tisserand, Robert and Balacs, Tony (1995) *Essential Oil Safety, A Guide for Health Professionals*, Churchill Livingstone

Valnet, Dr Jean (1991) *The Practice of Aromatherapy*, C.W. Daniel Company Ltd

Watt, Martin (1994) *Plant Aromatics*, private publication.

Wildwood, Chrissie (1996) *The Bloomsbury Encyclopaedia of Aromatherapy*, Bloomsbury

USEFUL ADDRESSES

ESSENTIAL OILS

New Horizon Aromatics
18 Obelisk Rd
Woolston
Southampton
SO19 9BN

Butterbur & Sage
7 Tessa Rd
Reading
Berkshire
RG1 8HH

Fragrant Earth Co Ltd
PO Box 182
Taunton
TA1 1YR

PROFESSIONAL JOURNALS

The Aromatherapy Quarterly
5 Ranelagh Avenue
London
SW13 0BY

The International Journal of Aromatherapy
PO Box 746
Hove
E. Sussex
BN3 3XA

PROFESSIONAL ASSOCIATIONS

The Federation of Holistic Therapists
38a Portsmouth Road
Woolston
Southampton
Hampshire
SO19 9AD

The Guild of Complementary Practitioners
Liddell House
Liddell Close
Finchampsted
Berkshire
RG40 4NS

The International Society of Professional Aromatherapists
c/o Hinckley and District Hospital
The Annex
Mount Rd
Hinckley
Leics
LE10 1AG

The International Federation of Aromatherapists
Stamford House
2–4 Chiswick High Rd
London
W4 1TH

GENERAL

The Aromatherapy Organisations Council (AOC)
3 Latymer Close
Braybrook
Market Harborough
Leicester
LE16 8LN
(representing 13 professional associations and 85 training establishments)

The Aromatherapy Trade Council (ATC)
PO Box 52
Market Harborough
Leicester
LE16 8ZX
(The aim of the ATC is to raise standards of quality and safety of Aromatherapy products.)

INDEX